AF839980

"*Clay Work and Body Image in Art Therapy* is an insightful synthesis of women's authentic expressions of body image experience and representation, with extensive theoretical integration and analysis. Trisha Crocker and Susan Carr present, through the art-based vignettes and the authors' reflective writing, a lyrical and clinical account of new knowledge in this field, emerging through the clay work sculptures. The book works on a number of levels – providing insight into the body image issues women face that echo and enrich our understanding, and how these issues can be passed down through the mother-daughter relationship. Offering new knowledge and a transparent process of analysis, this book is important reading for practicing therapists and students alike and sows the seed for further research in this important field."

Michal Bat-Or, *Art therapist, lecturer and researcher at University of Haifa, Israel*

"This well-researched book draws on the most helpful and influential theories which have become integral to UK art therapy practice: embodiment of emotions, attachment theory and the impact of the socio-cultural context on mental health and in this case, body-image. It elegantly demonstrates how clay has specific attributes which support the exploration of these issues within art therapy. Above all, it is anchored in the authors' extensive clinical experience and the stunning visual imagery makes it a much welcome publication which will be of interest to arts therapists, service users and artists in health."

Val Huet, PhD, *Director of Research & Development, British Association of Art Therapists*

Clay Work and Body Image in Art Therapy

Clay Work and Body Image in Art Therapy provides an important addition to resources available in the field of clay work and art therapy, highlighting the unique sensory aspects of the medium and its ability to provide a therapeutic resource for women who experience body image issues.

Chapters offer a comprehensive distillation of current knowledge in the field of body image, clay work, neuroscience, and art therapy, building a theoretical framework around personal narratives. Case studies examine the benefits of exploring body image through clay work within art therapy practice, providing a positive and contained way to find personal acceptance and featuring photographs of clay body image sculptures created by research participants that highlight their individual stories and experiences. As well as offering both clinical and practical implications, the text provides a full protocol for the research and evaluation methods carried out, enabling further replication of the intervention and research methods by other therapists.

This book highlights clay work as a significant resource for art therapists, arts in health practitioners, and counsellors, providing an emotive yet contained approach to the development of personal body image acceptance and self-compassion.

Trisha Crocker, PhD, is an art therapist working with at-risk children and women in private practice. She runs workshops in clay-making and body image from her pottery in Oxfordshire, England.

Susan M.D. Carr, PhD, is an artist, author, and art therapist in private practice, and currently co-Editor-in-Chief of the *International Journal of Art Therapy*. She has also developed and researched Portrait Therapy.

Clay Work and Body Image in Art Therapy

Using Metaphor and Symbolism to Heal

Trisha Crocker
Susan M.D. Carr

Routledge
Taylor & Francis Group
NEW YORK AND LONDON

First published 2021
by Routledge
605 Third Avenue, New York, NY 10158

and by Routledge
2 Park Square, Milton Park, Abingdon, Oxon, OX14 4RN

Routledge is an imprint of the Taylor & Francis Group, an informa business

© 2021 Trisha Crocker and Susan M.D. Carr

The right of Trisha Crocker and Susan M.D. Carr to be identified as authors of this work has been asserted by them in accordance with sections 77 and 78 of the Copyright, Designs and Patents Act 1988.

All rights reserved. No part of this book may be reprinted or reproduced or utilised in any form or by any electronic, mechanical, or other means, now known or hereafter invented, including photocopying and recording, or in any information storage or retrieval system, without permission in writing from the publishers.

Trademark notice: Product or corporate names may be trademarks or registered trademarks, and are used only for identification and explanation without intent to infringe.

Library of Congress Cataloging-in-Publication Data
Names: Crocker, Trisha, author. | Carr, Susan M. D., author.
Title: Clay work and body image in art therapy : using metaphor and symbolism to heal / Trisha Crocker, Susan Carr.
Description: New York : Routledge, 2021. | Includes bibliographical references and index.
Identifiers: LCCN 2020048563 (print) | LCCN 2020048564 (ebook) | ISBN 9780367564667 (hardback) | ISBN 9780367564650 (paperback) | ISBN 9781003097884 (ebook)
Subjects: LCSH: Body image. | Imagery (Psychology) | Self-perception. | Art therapy.
Classification: LCC BF697.5.B63 C77 2021 (print) | LCC BF697.5.B63 (ebook) | DDC 306.4/613—dc23
LC record available at https://lccn.loc.gov/2020048563
LC ebook record available at https://lccn.loc.gov/2020048564

ISBN: 978-0-367-56466-7 (hbk)
ISBN: 978-0-367-56465-0 (pbk)
ISBN: 978-1-003-09788-4 (ebk)

Typeset in Times New Roman
by Apex CoVantage, LLC

This book is dedicated to the 16 women who generously shared their body image stories and their sculptures during the PhD project, and for making this book possible, we thank you . . .

Contents

Figures

Chapter 1

Chapter 2

Chapter 4

Chapter 5

Chapter 6

Chapter 7

Chapter 8

Chapter 10

Acknowledgements

Trisha: I would like to thank my mother, who taught me that I could always do anything I wanted as long as I perservered and didn't give up. To Professor Mitchell J. Rycus, who encouraged me to begin the PhD and was always there for me with moral support to the very end and after. Lastly, I would like to thank my daughter Charlie MacGregor for her support and constant love throughout the long process of the PhD and the creation of the book. Charlie's photography of the women's images has enhanced the pages of the book. I would also like to dedicate Chapters 2 and 6, on Body Image and Mothers and Daughters, to my sister Ellen, who knows better than anyone the impact of a mother on a daughter's self-esteem. You were a driving force from day one of the PhD and were forever in my thoughts throughout the process.

Susan: It has been a great experience collaborating with Trisha on this book, and exciting to see it through to publication. As always, with any project there are people working quietly in the background that make it all possible and for whom thanks are in order. I would like to thank my partner Terry for all his support and endless good humour, despite me locking myself away in a garret room for months on end, especially as this coincided with a national lockdown due to the pandemic! I would also like to thank my Mum and Dad, and sons James and Matthew, for their on-going support for 'yet another project!'

Section 1

Preparing the Ground – *Digging for Clay*

1 Introduction and Context

Body Image, Art Therapy, and Clay Work

A Very Personal Journey, by Trisha Crocker

I was born in Hollywood, California and brought up in Beverly Hills during the 1950s, an area of the world known for its obsession with the 'perfect' body. Becoming a professional dancer in the 1960s, I attended many auditions where the choreographer was less interested in the perfect kick than in the perfect bottom! One can point the finger at social media, air-brushed models, even painfully thin Disney characters; whatever the reasons the results are the same – women feel pressurised to conform to an unrealistic female body image, and to feel flawed and ugly if they do not, resulting in a lack of self-esteem, and poor body image.

My personal interest in the effect of poor body image on women developed when, later in life, I became a dance and fitness instructor. I remember how astounded I was to find that so many of the beautiful women I taught had negative thoughts about their bodies. I was particularly concerned as these women seemed outwardly confident and comfortable in their bodies, and yet they all expressed stress and anxiety around their body image. I wondered why so many women seemed dissatisfied with their bodies, and where this self-judgement emanated from.

Later, from my experience as an art therapist working with women with a negative body image, I began to see how this could lead to the women experiencing feelings of utter despair and self-loathing, resulting in anxiety, depression, and a lack of self-confidence. I began thinking about the potential value of creating images using the tactile and three-dimensional properties of clay as a safe tactile material for women to explore their body image, and turn their negative experiences into positive ones.

I was also inspired to develop a suitable intervention for women with body image issues after reading a book called *A Waist Is a Terrible Thing to Mind* (Philips et al. 2000), a collection of poems and stories written by women across America, describing the ways in which they battled with a negative body image. I discovered the book quite unintentionally whilst exploring body image through working on my own series of clay sculptures of women. My attention was immediately seized by the urgency and despair in the writings, a despair I recognised in my own art therapy clients, underlining for me just how important this subject is. I was also struck by the link between mothers and daughters and body image. Here 'Maggie' writes about her anxiety for her unborn daughter:

> Most of all, this is for my daughter, a daughter who is not even born. A daughter I would comfort, tasting the tears off her cheek when one day she, too, learns that she is not pretty enough, she is not perfect enough [. . .] simply not enough.
>
> (Maggie, quoted in Philips et al. 2000, p.166)

Maggie goes on to say:

> This is for the tears I will cry with her because I have no words to feed the empty place in her that will never understand that she absolutely IS just enough.
>
> (ibid.)

Ideas for the intervention were sparked when, during a clay teaching session, I intuitively sculpted a small shape and gave it breasts and a belly. In between the weekly sessions I felt drawn back to the studio to make another, larger sculpture of a round-bellied women with full breasts and buttocks. When women from a ceramics class I was running at the time walked into my pottery the following week and saw the sculpture, one pointed at one of my sculptures and exclaimed "That is definitely me!" The following week another lady from the class walked in and saw my latest sculpture and exclaimed "This one is me!" I therefore became aware that women identified strongly with my sculptures, and I felt compelled to sculpt the female form in all its multitudes of shapes and sizes and at different ages. This resulted in a series of over 200 sculptures I called *An Army of Women* (see Figures 1 on p.5 & 2 on p.6), which were exhibited in 2008 at Norden Farm, in Maidenhead, The Mirror Gallery, South Hill Park, Bracknell, and the Henley Festival. *An Army of Women* spoke to me about feelings of 'solidarity' with all women and the idea of there being 'strength in numbers'. It seemed to me that each of my sculpted 'women' possessed a *soul* and a reason for existence, and the key message I wanted the *Army of Women* to portray, was for women to recognise that each of them, in their own unique way, is beautiful, and is 'enough', no matter what shape or size they are.

In a review written about the exhibition, Dr Outi Remes (2010) wrote that the work portrayed 'bodies of difference' and a 'celebration of the female form' with 'multiple body shapes and colours' without any hierarchy of race or class. At the exhibition, I witnessed strong emotions from many female visitors, who often remained near the sculpture they most identified with, seemingly searching for the 'soul' within the piece. Through this 'soul searching' they were able to find their own personal connections and interpretations within the 'army'.

Therefore, the *Army of Women* is testimony to my personal exploration of the female form in clay, something that has been explored as far back as

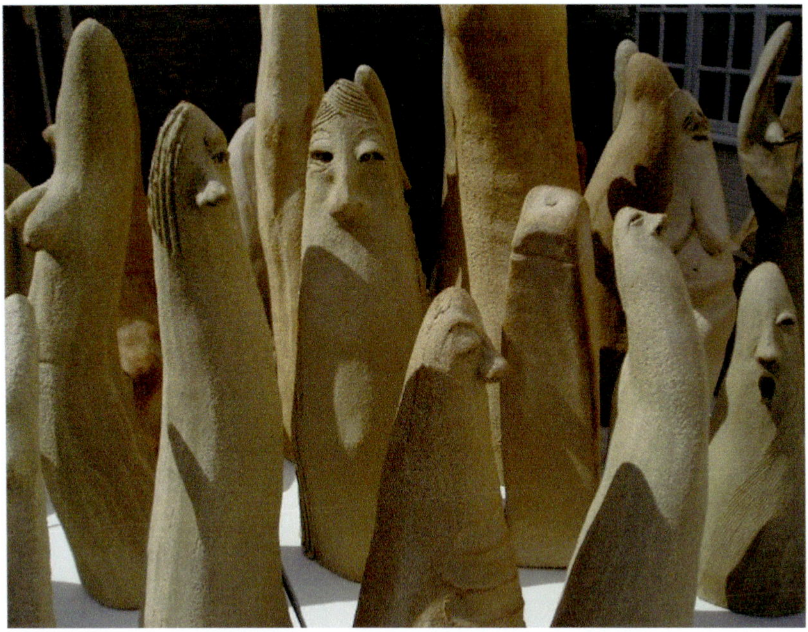

Figure 1 "An Army of Women No. 1" by Trisha Crocker, 2008.

28,000 years ago (Henley 2002), since humans first took a fist of clay or stone and fashioned it into the shape of a woman. Small figures, often referred to as 'Venuses' with overly large breasts and bellies, were fashioned out of clay, then placed on hot coals until they exploded, signifying their magical significance and power as objects of fertility (ibid., p.83). Clearly, despite the span of centuries, the female form remains a subject of curiosity and awe, and these ancient creations resonate and share a kinship with my own early clay work and those of the women who share their own personal stories and creations around body image within this book.

In my own art therapy practice I use a person-centred approach to clay work, with the focus often being on that of *play*. I currently work at a school with excluded children aged between 5 and 11 years, and *play* works because it comes naturally to children, and my role is about 'being with' the child, allowing them to interpret their creations, and develop personal understanding so that opportunities for change can become a natural outcome. This same paradigm of clay work as 'play' was used in the PhD research case studies (Crocker 2017), discussed in this book. Play speaks of letting go, of being given permission to 'make a mess', allowing a sense of freedom and learning to develop, within the 'held' therapeutic space. My PhD thesis explored clay as a tool to help women heal their body image issues, and the evidence provided by this is outlined within this book, offering a new intervention for art therapists to use in their practice, providing the full protocol and analysis techniques used within the study to aid replication. The evidence provided within this book

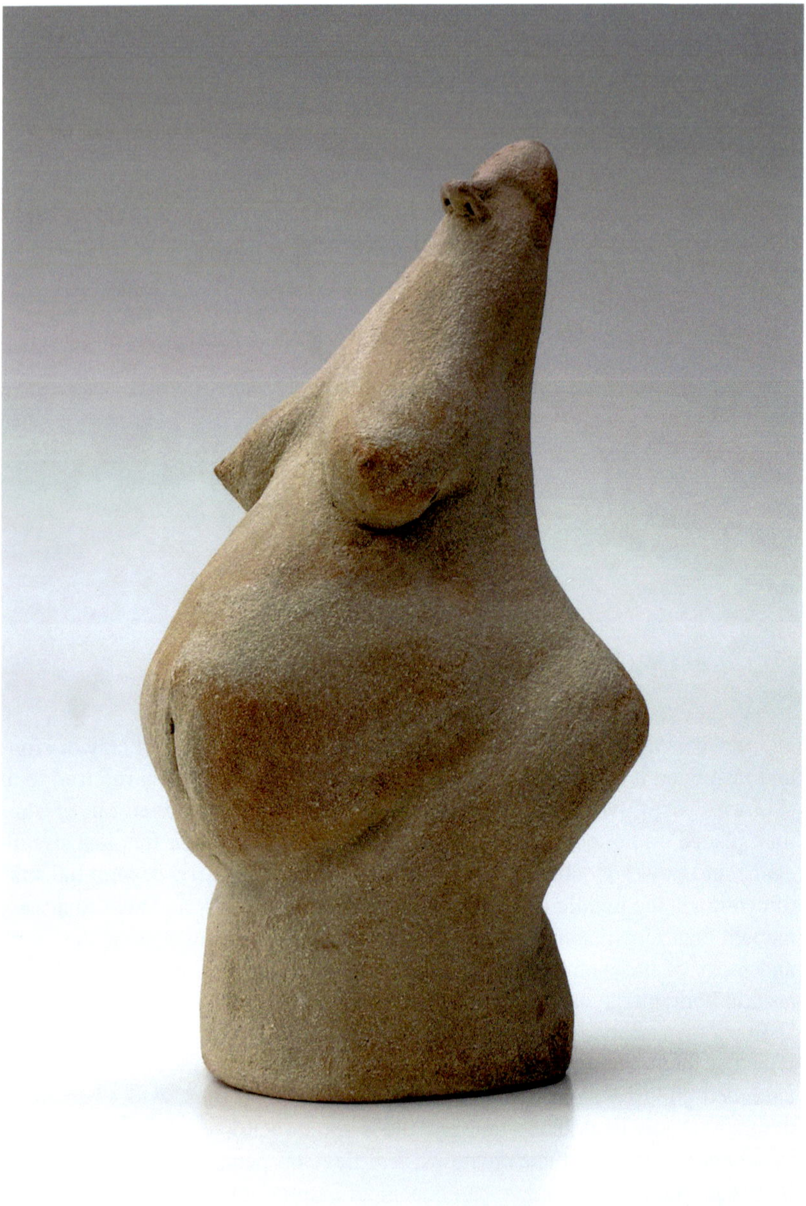

Figure 2 "Large and Lovely" by Trisha Crocker, 2008.

shows that women who create their body image in clay are (perhaps for the first time) able to take ownership of that image and to heal the psychological trauma of never feeling 'good enough'.

A Creative Collaboration: Embodiment and Self-Portrayal, by Susan Carr

It was a natural development for Trisha and I to collaborate on this book. When we were art therapy students together, we both aspired to continue our MA research by individually undertaking a PhD, and although the subject matter of our PhDs differ, they are linked by a fundamental interest in self-portrayal and disturbances in body image, whether it be through the impact of illness, or the impossibility of living up to idealistic female social stereotypes.

My own interest in body image was sparked by my work as an art therapist in the field of palliative care. My PhD – developing *Portrait Therapy* (2015, 2018) – was therefore inspired by working with clients, and involved developing an art therapy intervention for patients living with life threatening or chronic illnesses. *Portrait Therapy* reverses the traditional terms of engagement within art therapy and uses the art therapist's artistic practice or 'third hand' (Kramer 1971, 1977, 2000; Carr 2014, 2015, 2017, 2018) to create portraits *for* patients; however, in a series of 'negotiations', the patients co-design their own portraits – directing how they wish to be portrayed.

This builds on an understanding that severe illness is not just an attack on the body, it is an attack on a person's sense of self-identity and body image, shattering the means by which a person experiences the world, and by which they also are experienced. This profound sense of loss and disruption to self-identity and body image contributes to a person's sense of distress and powerlessness and is made manifest in statements such as "I don't know who I am anymore" and "I look in the mirror and say 'who's that?'"

As body image is an integral part of self-identity, it is important to explore this in relation to the creation of an 'embodiment' of the self in clay. Concepts such as 'self' and 'identity' have been historically, and to this day, a complex and contested phenomenon (Bauman 2004 p.77; Lawler 2008), with meanings that are both ambivalent and elusive (Vecchi 2004, p.2). However, they remain key topics of interest across the social sciences (e.g. Oyserman et al. 2012; Leary & Tangney 2012).

For the purposes of this book, we describe a 'cohesive sense of self-identity' as comprising: 'a realistic body image, subjective self-sameness, consistent attitudes, temporality, gender, authenticity, and ethnicity' (Akhtar & Samuel 1996). However, Palmer's (2007 [1998]) description of identity is also important as it brings together all the diverse cultural and nurturing elements that may make up a person's sense of self-identity. He describes identity as

> [. . .] an evolving nexus where all the forces that constitute my life converge in the mystery of self: my genetic makeup, the nature of the man and

> woman who gave me life, the culture in which I was raised, people who have sustained me and people who have done me harm, the good and ill I have done to others and to myself, the experience of love and suffering [. . .] identity is a moving intersection of the inner and outer forces that make me who I am, converging in the irreducible mystery of being human.
> (Palmer 2007 [1998], p.14)

Self-identities can therefore be viewed as relational and also culturally constructed (Evans 2005a, p.40) or at least culturally influenced, and as such characterised by change and fluidity, sometimes referred to as a 'reflexive project' (Giddens 1991, p. 32).

Embodiment

For renowned phenomenological philosopher Merleau-Ponty (1908–1961), the body is central to how we experience and interpret the world, and is the whole reason we have a world to experience (Merleau-Ponty 2002). Certainly, our embodiment is central to our experience as human beings and it is through our bodies that we are able to understand other people (ibid. p.186). This is something that Finlay (2009) describes as our 'embodied intersubjectivity', or our 'corporeal commonality' (p.8). As therapists and researchers, it is therefore important to be able to put 'oneself into the experience of the patient as much as possible, feeling it as if in one's own body – without losing a separate sense of self' (Yontef 2002, p.24).

With an understanding that the body or embodiment is central to all aspects of perception, consciousness, and human experience (Merleau-Ponty 2002), the concept of the body as *home* can be recognised, with body image sculptures therefore becoming a depiction of a person's sense of *homelike or unhomelike-being-in-the-world* (Svenaeus 2011). The idea of 'home' brings to mind a protective material environment, combining a sense of permanence, security and continuity, with a space that is full of emotional significance and meaning (Dupuis & Thorns 1998, p.30).

With our bodies so significant to our understanding of the world, it follows that as human beings we are intensely conscious of our own bodies and those of other people. A large part of the way we communicate with others is through body language or facial expressions, instantly recognising behavioural or emotional clues that tell us something about the thoughts, feelings and intended actions of the other person (Freeland 2010, p.154). When creating our own body image out of clay, the sculptural form becomes imbued with personal significance that can be perceived by others, it exists in space in a way that bodies do and has an intentionality that is recognisably human. This subject/object that is both 'me' and 'not me', 'home-like' and 'unhome-like', is a significant therapeutic vessel for exploring the intra-personal relationship one has with one's own body, and how that body relates to others and the world. The process of creating one's body image in clay enables people to depict themselves as they see themselves, through the lens of the distorted mirror that encapsulates all the damaging things others have said about their bodies over time, and then gradually rectify these distortions through the malleability of clay, coming to a more balanced and personally healing view of the self.

Clay as a Therapeutic Medium

For most of the women who attended the body image sessions featured in this book, clay work was new to them, or at the very least a distant memory from art classes at school, or from making 'mud pies' in the garden as a child. As such it was still a familiar material, something that was unlikely to provoke anxiety as a medium. Derived from the very building blocks of mother nature and the universe, the therapeutic and cathartic nature of clay is clearly evident, and the sensory playful qualities it exudes are plain to see.

In its natural form clay is: tactile, wet, malleable and messy, it can be shaped, scraped, cut, rolled, squashed, squeezed and even poured and 'clay has the capacity to be done and undone multiple times, providing the opportunity to smash down or remake a clay-sculpture' (Rubin 1984, p.58). Once fired, clay becomes solid, immovable, durable, and yet retains a fragility that reflects the human condition. The firing process, like that of life, is dangerous and unpredictable, with clay sculpture prone to breaking, cracking, or exploding within the kiln.

Clay is a sensory, tactile, three-dimensional material for creating one's own body image; it allows for play and reflection in ways that other two-dimensional materials do not. It can be cut, pulled apart and then repaired and put back together, becoming a metaphor for injury, trauma, and making whole again. These processes of change are the practical benefits of clay work. Within this context we understand the term 'clay work' (which other authors may write as 'clay-work' or 'claywork') to mean 'the process of handling, manipulating, and sculpting clay, and the products of these activities' (Sholt & Gavron 2006, p.66), highlighting that an 'art expression is not merely the final product but is also the process by which the product has been developed, and that process and product foster significant psychological processes, revealing meaningful information about the creators' inner world' (ibid.). In her therapeutic clay work with children, Rhodes (2008) suggests that pinching, poking, squeezing, constructing, and cutting away are what create the clay work.

A useful theory for therapeutic clay work was identified by Souter-Anderson (2010) as a *theory of contact: physical, emotional, and metaphorical;* she describes this as follows:

> [. . .] playing with the medium is a physical contact, a sensate experience, with the substance that appears to stir feelings and make contact with emotions whilst simultaneously engaging with the world, the imagination, thus incorporating a metaphorical contact.
>
> (Souter-Anderson 2010, p.51)

For the purposes of this book, and the research it refers to, we use Sholt and Gavron's (2006) description of the characteristics of 'clay work' as including 'procedural expression through touch, movement, and the three-dimensional aspect, the reflection of construction and deconstruction processes, and the regression process' (p.66). Sholt & Gavron also suggest that clay is 'a familiar material in art therapy and in psychotherapy' which many promote for its capacity to provide a therapeutic tool 'in individual and group therapies' (Sholt & Gavron 2006, p.66).

Working with clay stimulates all the senses and involves 'very primary forms of expression and communication' (Snir & Regev 2013, p.95). Henley (2002, p.75) believes that re-creating the body image in clay 'naturally invites projective identification into the art process' and suggests that the processes of creation and destruction inherent within clay work can be beneficial to clients. The clay sculpture can also be revisited over time, and held by the maker both figuratively and literally, as a reminder of change. Rabinor and Bilich (2002) suggest that clay work in art therapy, can be used to help clients change or adapt their body image (p.474). Cash and Pruzinsky (2002a) believe that non-clinical populations of women who experience negative body image could be helped with an experiential approach.

The beauty of working with clay is the direct, physical, and therefore sensory, contact the clients have with the art material. For Ogden (1989) human experience often relates to primitive experience, which may be dominated by the sensory experiences of touch and rhythm. The physical presence and materiality of clay sculptures mean that they can also be used as significant objects within rites and rituals. Cohen and Mills (1999) suggest that 'drawings, paintings and sculpture made in art therapy can reveal distorted body-image and introduce it into therapeutic conversation in a way that clients can tolerate' (p.204).

Art Therapy and Clay Work: Reviewing the Literature

The British Association of Art Therapists (BAAT) describes art therapy as:

> [. . .] a form of psychotherapy that uses art media as its primary mode of expression and communication. Within this context, art is not used as a diagnostic tool but as a medium to address emotional issues, which may be confusing and distressing.
>
> (BAAT 2004)

Art therapy is an accessible therapy, in that no skills in art are required, with the focus being mainly on what the art product represents or reveals about emotional or psychological issues.

Art therapy helps clients to bring to the surface and externalise issues which may have been internalised over many years, within a safe and contained environment. The therapeutic 'triangular relationship' (Schaverien 2000, p.55) between the art therapist, the client, and the art object, is an important aspect of art therapy theory, and it is therefore the presence of the *art object*, created by the client, that makes art therapy unique. Maintaining client/therapist boundaries is essential within art therapy in order to provide a safe space for clients to work freely with the art materials, explore their thoughts and feelings, and promote healing.

Research into art therapy as a therapeutic discipline has been ongoing since art therapy was developed during the 1940s in the UK by British artists and early art therapy pioneers – Edward Adamson (1911–1996) and Adrian Hill (1895–1977). Adamson and Hill were founder members of the British Association of Art Therapists (BAAT), established in 1964, with Hill becoming its first president (Ostrowska 2013; Hogan 2001).

It is not generally known that the use of clay and ceramics has its roots in the very inception of art therapy in the United Kingdom (SLaM 2018). One of the first documented instances of clay or ceramics being used is the presence of 500 ceramics, some dated 1948 (SLaM 2018), stored at the South London and Maudsley NHS Trust as part of the Edward Adamson collection. The collection as a whole consists of 5500 objects, including paintings, drawings, ceramics, sculptures and works in stone, flint and bone, that were created between 1946 and 1981, by in-patients at the long-stay mental health hospital, Netherne, where Adamson worked (ibid.).

Adamson's style was 'non-interventionalist', meaning he was against the psychological interpretation of patients' artwork, which he dismissed as 'the therapist's own projections', maintaining that only the creator of the work could explain their own image (O'Flynn 2011, pp.46–53). Adamson saw himself less as a 'therapist' but more as an 'artist' facilitator, with a broadly humanistic theoretical base (Ostrowska 2013), and an intermediary between the patients and the medical staff. The space within which Adamson worked was always called the *art studio* rather than a *therapeutic space* (Adamson 1970). Adamson is reported as saying

> [t]he actual 'therapy' is purely incidental. The important thing is the art [. . .] that's the thing that is getting them better. The mere fact that they put their brush to paper and try and paint.
>
> (Adamson, cited in Seftel 1987, p.50)

Adamson is also quoted as saying: 'The strength of the art therapist is in being an artist' (Seftel 1987, p.48). However, both Hill and Adamson became increasingly unhappy as the profession developed toward a psychodynamic and psychoanalytical orientation of art therapy (Hogan 2001), feeling that it was losing its focus on the *creation of art* as a fundamental aspect of healing in *art* therapy, with Adamson deciding to focus much more on *Outsider Art* (Ostrowska 2013). Adamson exhibited the collection in various galleries during his lifetime, including major international exhibitions of Outsider Art, with a view to reducing the stigma associated with mental health problems, by educating the public and highlighting through the art, the humanity and creativity of his patients (ibid.).

Art therapists use many different theoretical approaches when working with clients, e.g. humanistic and client-centred (Rogers 2003 [1951]) and existential (Yalom 1980) at one end of the theoretical continuum, and psychodynamic (Freud 1913 [1899]) and psychoanalytic (Jung 1933; Klein 1952) at the other. Many therapists use a variety of different approaches depending upon the client group and/or issues clients present. Similarly, the art materials used may be influenced by the client group or issues being addressed, with clay work being particularly recommended for art therapy work with children who have experienced abusive relationships. The research discussed within this book also indicates that clay is a useful medium for art therapy with women to explore body image issues.

Art therapy as a profession continues to develop theoretically and practically, with ongoing research in all areas of the discipline (e.g. research published within: *The International Journal of Art Therapy; Art Therapy: The Journal of the American Art Therapy Association*; *The Arts in Psychotherapy;* and the *Canadian Art Therapy Association Journal*. Clay work in art therapy practice is currently an under-researched area of practice, and therefore this book, and the PhD thesis from which the case studies are drawn, seek to address this balance, particularly addressing the area of clay work, women, and body image.

Clay Work in Art Therapy

> As an art therapy intervention, working with clay typically involves the shaping and manipulating of the material with the goal of producing a product where both the process of creating and the product are considered to hold significance for the interior world of the creator.
>
> (Henley 2002 p.23)

Whilst there is a general paucity of published research on the use of clay in art therapy, significant books have been written on the subject. Australian psychotherapist and educator Dr Patricia Sherwood developed a specific therapeutic discipline called 'Clay Therapy' (2004), from which she has written a book by the same name. Whilst this is not the same as using clay within the specific discipline of *art therapy*, Sherwood's work offers considerable insight into the use of clay to help clients with anger, grief, and related issues. Sherwood talks of the undiscovered potential of clay used in therapy, saying 'clay work is like the Cinderella of the art therapies' still waiting for her 'magic, her beauty and her ability to transform the wells of human suffering into places of insight and celebration' (Sherwood 2004, p.5).

Art therapist and educator Dr David Henley has written extensively on art therapy, and in 2002 wrote his book *Clayworks in Art Therapy*. As a ceramicist Henley speaks from experience when he talks about clay's potential for therapeutic application. In his book Henley uses case studies and vignettes to explore the theories, techniques and history of clay work and its power to enable positive therapeutic outcomes. By promoting both aesthetics and artistic integrity, Henley offers a holistic approach to working therapeutically with clay.

In Lynn Souter-Anderson's (2010) book *Touching Clay, Touching What? The Use of Clay in Therapy*, she takes an existential theoretical stance, focusing on what it means to be human, and how clay work can enable the release of emotions, memories and sensations, that can be explored within a safe therapeutic space. Souter-Anderson outlines a sound theoretical basis for the use of clay in therapy, based on her own original research, and her deep understanding of the processes involved. Writing of the lack of research into clay work, Souter-Anderson says, 'The value and particularly the therapeutic significance of using clay in therapy has essentially not been recognised or understood' (2010, pp.11–13).

Art therapist Cornelia Elbrecht (2013) writes about a technique she has developed for using clay with clients, something she has defined as the 'Clay Field'®; Elbrecht describes this as 'a rectangular box filled with non-gritty clay' (2013, p.19), and as a 'psycho-physiological art therapy process that engages the hands with the material of clay within the safe setting of a containing box', and includes 'an intricate interaction between human neurobiology and expressions of lived experiences' (ibid.). In a later article on the 'Clay Field'® Elbrecht and Antcliff (2014) suggest that 'haptic perception allows non-verbal access to psychological and sensorimotor processes thwarted by trauma' and that trauma can be resolved via touch (p.19).

Creating a three-dimensional object out of clay within a safe therapeutic space has many advantages; for Jung (1916, p.82), giving personal disturbances or issues a 'visible shape' produces a 'vitalising influence', something that enables the issues/disturbances to be reproduced in either a concrete or symbolic form. The three-dimensional process of forming the female figure in clay enables clients to turn the image around 360 degrees and view it from different directions and angles (Buchalter 2004; Henley 2002). This allows one to look at the figure as a whole and from different perspectives, unlike the two-dimensionality of drawing or painting, which allows viewing from just one direction.

In her book *Women Who Run with the Wolves* (1992) American poet, psychoanalyst and post-trauma specialist, Clarissa Pinkola Estes states: 'It is clear that the instinctive nature of women values body and spirit far more for their ability to be vital, responsive, and enduring than by any measure of appearance' (p.199). She goes on to say that

> [d]estroying a woman's instinctive affiliation with her natural body cheats her of confidence. It causes her to perseverate about whether she is a good person or not and bases her self-worth on how she looks instead of who she is.
>
> (p.201)

Cohen and Mills (1999) suggest that 'when clients believe there is something deeply wrong with their body, they might also need to defend against this belief by dissociating (the mind is me, the body is not-me)' (p.203). The sensory nature of clay and its capacity to be 'body-like' (Foster 1997, p.68) means that it can 'stimulate life-like perception' (Waldman 1997, p.12), serving as a 'bridge between the sensory experiences imprinted in the body and conscious awareness of these events' (ibid.). Ellis (1989) also suggests that the use of clay in therapeutic encounters encourages client reflection, through its tactile qualities, and can enable the reflection of unconscious bodily experiences, through embodied actions such as stroking, stabbing, smoothing, and squashing (p.267).

In her art therapy case study using clay to help a female client ('Susan') diagnosed with depression, Waldman (1999) considers how the social construction of gender, and the demands put on women, is linked to the prevalence of depression in women (p.10). The case study describes how using clay was significant in enabling 'Susan' to 'access memories of childhood trauma and to develop a more authentic subjectivity' (ibid.). Waldman also suggests that working with clay in therapy can be a 'powerful medium to engage clients physically by stimulating primary sensory experience, directing them to expel rage and experiment with being in control' (ibid.).

In their review of clay work in art therapy and psychotherapy Sholt and Gavron (2006) suggest that, [. . .] 'the development of the ability for three-dimensional representation in clay has not received enough attention' and that further research in this important area is required (p.67). The therapeutic research within this book is therefore, in part, a response to the calls for further research in the use of clay within art therapy (Sholt & Gavron 2006; Henley 2002; Golomb and McCormick 1995; and Woltmann 1993, p.66). Clearly a wider understanding of the process and product of clay work in art therapy is necessary to develop an understanding of its potential therapeutic use and the nature of any risks or ethical considerations posed by this medium.

In a review of 35 clinical reports Sholt & Gavron (2006) identified six main therapeutic factors of clay work in art therapy and psychotherapy; these include facilitating: 'expression of emotions'; 'catharsis'; 'rich and deep expressions'; 'verbal communication'; 'revealing unconscious material'; and 'concretisation and symbolisation: The embodiment of inner representations in visual images' (ibid. p.70). The benefits for clients offered by clay work include 'a significant exploration of self by clients and therapists that enable the detection and integration of primal experiences of the self, and its multifaceted nature. It is by which clients widen their access to their inner selves and thus continue their journey of becoming' (Sholt & Gavron 2006, p.71).

The therapeutic nature of clay and clay work within therapy is inherent within the three-dimensional nature of clay and the opportunity for clients to create a concrete three-dimensional object, which can become a symbol and metaphor for their own inner world and experiences (Sholt & Gavron 2006, p.68). The three-dimensionality of clay means that it can closely resemble, recreate, and represent objects from real life (Sholt & Gavron 2006, p.68). It can also be used to create figures that represent powerful emotions that were previously inaccessible to clients (Henley 2002; Mciver 2001; Brock 1991; Keyes 1984; Mitchell 1984).

There is evidence within the literature of a connection between loss and clay work. Henley (2002) investigates clay and 'object loss' in his art therapy work with a young teenage girl whose mother had died, saying the girl felt unable to talk about her grief. However, after a few months of therapy, the girl created a large clay cup on which she scratched the word 'Mother'; the girl loved to hold this cup and through this she was able to begin to talk about how much she missed her mother's touch (Henley 2002). This demonstrates the potential for clay to be used to help clients who are experiencing loss and mourning, using created objects, or the created image of a lost loved one as a way to cope with emotional pain. For Henley (1991), the malleability of clay and the manipulation it can withstand in a therapeutic setting are important aspects of its therapeutic value, as he says: 'Clay taps into the depths of human consciousness. [. . .]. Clay's plastic, malleable nature gave birth to the metaphor that it possesses a life and body of its own' (p.67).

Research has shown that clay work can empower the creators (Snir & Regev 2013). Snir & Regev (2013) write of the findings from their research, claiming that working with clay enabled clients to report a sense of 'relief', 'release', and a 'sense of calm' (p.98). With reference to their clients' use of clay they maintain that 'childhood memories evoked by working with clay were particularly prominent' and that the sensual property of clay brought forth 'memories of smells, touch and baking bread' (pp.98–99).

It is important to keep in mind the interaction that can happen between the art materials offered and the particular characteristics of the client/artist (Snir & Regev 2013; Moon 2010; Sholt & Gavron 2006). This holds particular relevance for clinicians who offer art therapy to clients with specific physical and emotional needs (Snir & Regev 2013, p.100). The versatility of clay as a therapeutic material is beneficial as it can either be worked upon and left unfinished, or it can be painted/glazed and fired (Yaretzky & Levinson 1996, quoted in Abramowitz 2013, p.2). Glazing a finished piece such as a cup or bowl can make it waterproof. Also, if a client decides to glaze and fire a piece, they can then choose to display it in their home, which can create further opportunities for self-reflection.

Art therapists including Elbrecht 2013; Elbrecht & Antcliff 2014; Sholt and Gavron 2006; O'Brien 2004; Fabre-Lewin 1997; McNiff 1992; and Ellis 1989, have written about the haptic qualities of specific three-dimensional art materials used by clients in therapeutic sessions, e.g. making a 'mess' by rubbing hands into paint, scrunching and ripping paper, rubbing wool into felt, and specifically clay work. Henley (2002) and Sholt and Gavron (2006), believe that the use of clay in art therapy can be a sensory, whole-body experience for the client, an experience that can lead to moments of 'illumination' (Malchiodi

1998, pp.66–68) or 'breakthrough' experiences, where one achieves a discovery or 'is satisfied with what one has created' (ibid.).

Sensory three-dimensional art materials such as clay involve the haptic processes of touch, sight, smell, and sound. Because of clay's 'body-likeness' some clients may find it stimulates a perception of being life-like (Foster 1997) containing uncomfortable feelings, and therefore can act as 'a bridge between *sensory* experiences imprinted in the body and conscious awareness of these events' (Waldman 1999, p.12). However, clay work in particular also involves what is often called a 'sixth sense', that of *proprioception* (also known as kinaesthesis), which is a sense of body position or movement that 'combines with other senses to locate external objects relative to the body and contributes to body image' (Taylor 2009, p.1143–1149).

Art therapist Arthur Robbins (1999) talks about how working in clay helped him to discover his 'soul in the mess', and that it '[. . .] seemed to touch such a deep part of me, creating such a sense of excitement and aliveness that I could hardly wait from one class to another' (p.121). In a qualitative study on the use of clay in a psychiatric day hospital in Brazil, A.H. de Morais et al. (2014) conclude that 'the use of clay as a therapeutic method by psychiatric patients promoted creativity, self-consciousness, and benefited those who sought anxiety relief' (p.128).

The properties of clay mean it has a unique capacity to reflect bodily experiences that are unconscious, through the tactile and versatile nature of the medium (Ellis 1989). Clay can be a powerful medium for clients, in that it engages them physically, stimulating often primary sensory experience, meaning they can safely expel anger, and experiment with being in 'control' (Waldman 1999, p.12). As such clay modelling can help clients to tell stories about attachment, and also self-harm and destruction (Gampel 1993, p.289), as well as 'bypass intellectual defences, invite playfulness' and 'confront distorted body imagery' (Waldman, 1999, p.12). Art therapist Judith Waldman (ibid.) discusses a case study where changing the art materials offered to a client to clay, changed the course of therapy, with her client 'Susan' explaining that, with clay, "I express more of my basic feelings with it. It's not just cosmetic and pretty. I'm more involved."

This book, and the thesis from which the case studies are drawn, fills a gap in the available research and literature on the specific subject of clay as an art therapy intervention for women exploring issues related to body image. Art therapy sourcebooks/handbooks (e.g. Malchiodi 1998; Case & Dalley 2000) have been remiss in referencing clay as an art therapy material in the subject indexing. It is difficult to understand why such a versatile, sensory, and healing art material should be side-lined in this way. There are reasons that make clay a more difficult material to work with, e.g. these are: a lack of knowledge around using clay; the cost of the materials and access to a kiln; health and safety issues; the storage of 3D sculptures; and the need for an art studio where the 'mess' created by clay can be contained and accommodated. Whilst these are significant issues, the benefits of overcoming them, to enable clients with specific issues to work in this way, are clear.

The Power of Clay Work: Ethical Considerations

Rubin (in Snir and Regev, 2013, p.100) writes of how important it is for art therapists to have an in-depth knowledge of the art materials they offer to clients within therapy sessions. As Malchiodi (quoted in Snir and Regev, 2013 p.94) says:

> Our understanding of the therapeutic potential of each [art] material and its unique "personality" is significant to the ability to design suitable interventions for clients.

This is specifically important when offering clay, as it has sensual as well as tactile qualities, which can be enjoyable for clients, however, its messiness and wetness may bring up unconscious material (Kagin & Lusebrink, 1978, quoted in Sholt & Gavron 2006, p.71), as well as unwelcome memories or feelings of disturbance for the client. Kramer and Schehr (1983) suggest that 'clay invites regression' and can result in 'playful behaviour that easily takes on an oral, anal, phallic or genital character', which can lead to the integration of fragmented parts of the self into sculptural works that contain the whole (p.77). Enabling abused children to work in clay can help children to open up about their abuse, either during, or after, the clay work took place (Kramer 2000).

Strong emotional responses to clay work are therefore important to consider when working with clients (Henley 2002), in particular clay's 'propensity to loosen controls given its faecal, smearing qualities and its dirtiness, which can rekindle early psychosexual conflicts' (Schlossberg 1983, p.103). Regressive work can be anxiety provoking for clients, therefore extreme care should be taken by therapists to ensure that a client is ready for this kind of work and able to withstand the emotional impact.

The intensity of clay work and its propensity to bring up unconscious material means caution should be used when working with art therapy clients who have experienced abuse or trauma (Sholt & Gavron 2006, p.71). Rhodes (2008) states that 'the clay therapist must always be ready to step in to shore up weak psychic structure and collapsing pieces' (p.27). Creating images in clay can be challenging, perhaps also due to the fragility of clay when dry (Sholt & Gavron 2006).

The fragility of clay can be a negative aspect of the process, but it can also be turned into a positive, as Yalom (2003, p.36) advises: 'Recall the fundamental therapy principle that all that happens is grist for the mill.' Therefore, if when firing, a piece cracks, or breaks off, or if the entire piece explodes in the kiln, this can be used by the therapist to help the client explore important metaphors around loss, damage, breaking, fragility, impermanence, incompleteness, imperfection, and death, as well as repair, renewal and recovery, particularly if a process of *visible mending* (Jones 2008; Carr 2015) is utilised.

Clay work as Meaningful Play

> Play lies at the core of creativity and innovation.
>
> (Brown & Vaughan 2009, pp.4–5)

Play is an important, pleasurable activity that enlivens, energises and eases depressed mood, promoting a sense of optimism and creativity (Brown & Vaughan 2009, pp.4–5). Infants begin to play very early on, as a way to make sense of their bodies and surroundings (ibid. p.83). Neuroscientists, biologists, social scientists, psychologists, and researchers recognise that play is a 'profound biological process' that has evolved over millennia to promote survival in many animal species (ibid. p.4). In higher animals, play fosters empathy, and enables complex social groups to be formed, and of all the animal species it is humans that play the most (ibid. p.5). Human beings are 'built to play and built through play', it is the 'purest expression of our humanity, the truest expression of our individuality' (ibid.).

According to Winnicott, play is vitally important in the development of self-identity; he describes it as a place where a person is able to *find* one's self. He says that 'it is in playing and only in playing that the individual child or adult is able to be creative and to use the whole personality, and it is only in being creative that the individual discovers the self (Winnicott 1971a, p.54).

Unfortunately, at some point as children grow into adulthood, they are made to feel guilty about playing, and told that it is *childish* or a *waste of time* (Brown & Vaughan 2009), and they are therefore *shamed* into giving it up (ibid. p.145). Creating a play space through building sculptures in clay can therefore help clients to reconnect to their 'inner child' (Carr 2017), where memories of making mud pies, modelling animals and figures in Plasticine®, Play-Doh® or pastry, come to the fore, and they are once again given *permission* to *play*.

Play, and art therapy as a 'play space', are therefore key theoretical constructs used within clay work, which happen within the 'transitional space' between the therapist and client. When clients are unable to 'play' or use the art materials, then the therapist will help the client relearn this skill (Winnicott 1968, pp.711–716). Winnicott (1896–1971) described 'transitional space' as:

> [. . .] a space between inner and outer worlds, which is also the space between people – the transitional space – [within which] intimate relationships and creativity occur.
>
> (Winnicott 1953, p.89)

In art therapy this 'held space' has also been described as a 'framework for freedom' that is both a 'physical and psychological space in which it is safe to be freely creative' (Rubin 2001 p.25) and to play.

Betensky (1995) claims that when using clay in therapy, the initial 'pre-art play' is a time for experimenting with the materials, and can last for anything from a few minutes to a few sessions, depending on the needs of the client (p.15). This initial phase ends when the client begins to invest meaning in the object they are creating, and they are able to describe it to the therapist (ibid.). Play can therefore be seen as a crucial stage of therapy, a time for the client to connect with the material and feel a sense of *held freedom to create* within the physical and psychological space created by the therapist (Crocker 2017, p.58).

The play space is also a space for the body, where physical activity can be safely explored and enacted. Therefore, clay work provides this physical space for the body, to move and to experiment and – as discussed in Chapter 3 – through the mirror neuron process clients are also able to physically experience or copy in their minds the movements and actions of others as they also work on their body image sculptures.

Play that uses movement, such as clay work, 'lights up the brain and fosters learning, innovation, flexibility, adaptability, and resilience' (Brown & Vaughan 2009, p.84). Play also seems to be important for health, as REM sleep and play 'share similar brain stem evolutionary biological patterns' (Brown & Vaughan 2009, p.204). This indicates that the need for play may be linked to the vital human requirement for rest and renewal (Medic et al. 2017).

> What's shocking is the similarity between the biological need for play and our body's need for rest, a topic that also emerged as a major theme in Wholehearted living. It seems that living and loving with our whole hearts requires us to respect our bodies' need for renewal. When I first researched the ideas of rest, sleep, and sleep debt—the term for not getting enough—I couldn't believe some of the consequences of not getting proper rest.
>
> (Brown, 2010, pp.227–228).

A biological and psychological need for play means that 'the opposite of play is not work – the opposite of play is depression' (Brown, quoted in Brown 2010, p.101). Getting play right can enhance all areas of a person's life, it can help provide joy and insight and 'the irony to deal with paradox, ambiguity, and fatalism' (Brown & Vaughan 2009, p.202). However, Brown and Vaughn warn that 'advanced play' can cause pain and discomfort as well as pleasure (ibid. p.205); it is therefore not always easy, but is a vital component in exploring the self (ibid. p.212).

2 The Distorted Mirror

Body Image, the Critical Mother, and Shame

This chapter is based on the premise that body image and the way we see ourselves – both physically and as an aspect of our self-identity, is built from our earliest experience of interpersonal relationships and a comparison of ourselves to other people in the wider world (Tantleef-Dunn and Gokee 2002, p.108; Frank 1997; Grytten & Måseide 2006; Wright 2009), and also through the influence of culture and the media. One of the first to write about the relational nature of body image was Paul Schilder (1950), when he argued that body image is not just something a person creates through seeing themselves in a mirror or photographs, but is also a reflection of the interactions and attitudes of other people to our body. Schilder was also interested in how a personal body image was not always a 'true' reflection of that person's size or shape (ibid.), something which will be discussed further in chapter 3.

Body Image

Many contemporary artists have explored, and become preoccupied with, personal and generic issues around the theme of the body or body image in their artwork (e.g. Orlan, Anthony Gormley, Tracey Emin, Marina Abramovich, etc.). Exhibitions such as Julie Bartholemew's *Transitional Bodies* (2006) tell the story of living in a consumer culture where women are encouraged to change their bodies through invasive interventions such as plastic surgery, or through gruelling diet and exercise in order to fit into a perceived idealistic, normalised and (for most) unreachable body image.

Other artists, such as Cheryl-Ann Webster seek to counteract this view. In her (2006) exhibition entitled *The Beautiful Women Project*, she displayed 120 life-sized sculptures of women's torsos, revealing the varied busts and midriffs of women aged 19–91 years, that were decorated to reflect an aspect of each woman's life-journey. Webster writes that the project was created as a way to help audiences 'to compare reality with socially-created, unattainable images of beauty, portrayed in our culture' (Webster 2006, p.1).

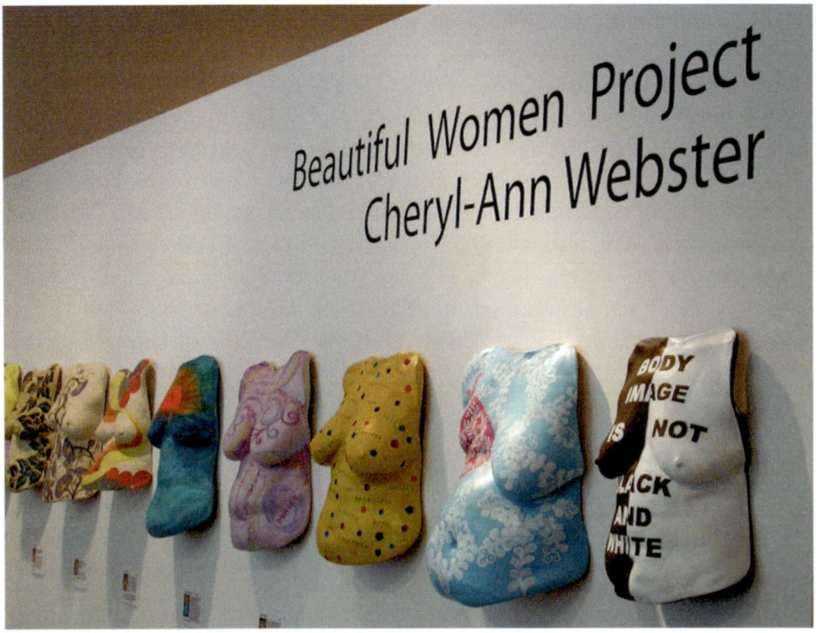

Figure 3 "The Beautiful Women Project" by Cheryl-Ann Webster, 2006.

As Webster says:

> Our bodies tell our life story. They are portraits of our journeys and experiences. Knowing that our body is beautiful just as it exists is a message more people need to see and hear.
>
> (Webster, 2006, p.1)

The term *body image* is a complex and contested one, and its meaning changes depending upon the discipline within which it is discussed (Cash 2004), however, for the purpose of this book we will use Grogan's (2008) description of body image as 'a person's perceptions, thoughts, and feelings about his or her body' (p.3) as this includes a person's psychological perceptions and attitudes they may have to their own body, as well as their experience of embodiment (ibid.). Many different words can be used to describe issues people experience with their own body image, e.g. appearance dissatisfaction, size perception inaccuracy, body dysmorphia, body dysphoria, body concern, body distortion, body image disturbance and body image disorder. However, the focus of the case studies contained within this book was not to diagnose or label disturbances found in an individual, but to enable clients to use clay as a way to explore their own body image and find a new level of personal understanding and self-acceptance.

Issues with body image are not a new phenomenon. Fisher and Cleveland (1968) published their book *Body image and Personality* over 50 years ago, and the issues raised remain as valid today as they did half a century ago, if anything the situation has been exacerbated by access to social media and advertising campaigns that include ultra-thin models, and children's toys (such as Barbie dolls) with impossibly tiny waists. The focus in advertising on body imperfections on the one hand, and the promotion of 'airbrushed' 'perfect' bodies on the other, clearly contributes to an increase in negative body image and disordered eating, with an increase in the diagnosis of eating disorders over the past 20 years (Galmiche et al. 2019), especially in children and young adults (Morris & Katzman 2003). Naturally this has become a matter of concern, and therefore research has focused specifically within this area i.e. obesity and anorexia nervosa, meaning that body image issues for women who don't fall into these extreme categories has been less researched (Schwartz & Brownell 2002, p.206). However, women in general are under constant pressure from advertising to look a certain way, and to feel inadequate, ugly, and inferior if they do not.

The visual nature of clay body image sculpture engages with our human need to present ourselves visually to others, and their ability to depict ambiguity, emotion and tacit knowledge through metaphor and symbolism is an important way they work. The gift of vision is wonderfully complicated, and those who study it are just beginning to understand what it involves. However, over 150 years ago Florence Nightingale understood the capacity for 'beauty' or aesthetically empathic images and objects to move and heal, both mentally and physically. She said:

> The effect in sickness of beautiful objects, and especially of brilliancy of colour is hardly appreciated at all. [. . .] People say the effect is only on the mind. It is no such thing. The effect is on the body, too. As little as we know about the way in which we are affected by form, by colour and light, we do know this, that they have an actual physical effect. [. . .] Variety of form and brilliance of colour in the objects presented to the patients is an actual means of recovery.
>
> (Nightingale, 1992 [1860], p.81)

'Beauty' is often described as a 'universal need of human beings', which 'brings consolation in sorrow and affirmation in joy', and something that shows human life to be 'worthwhile' (Scruton 2009). Beauty is said to be in the eye of the beholder and therefore entirely subjective, however, the effect of the media's preoccupation with an idealised version of beauty as 'perfection' is arguably a damaging one. A healthier vision of beauty is that found in Japanese *Wabi-Sabi,* which is described as 'a beauty of things imperfect, impermanent, and incomplete' (Koren 1998, p.7), which can also be described as *aesthetic resonance* (Carr 2015, p.224) – a 'process of adding beauty, complexity and coherence through many layered meanings' within self-images (ibid.). Aesthetics can also promote a sense of meaning through adding *coherence* to something *discordant* (Carr 2015, p.224), as Dissanayake says:

> Another way of looking at it is to recognize that meaning is aesthetic. Ordinary day-to-day life is formless, incoherent. When shaped and embellished or transformed as in ritual or play or art it takes on a greater or more significant reality so that when we find something to have coherence it seems to be 'aesthetic'. When we feel something to be aesthetic we recognize that it is coherent.
>
> (1980, p.404)

Creating body image sculptures as self-portraits, is part of the historic tradition of human representation and display, something which performs an important component of being human (Freeland 2010, pp.190–191). However, there is a difference between what we 'say in constituting ourselves and what we actually do when we go out and show ourselves to others in the world' (ibid.). This difference is characterised by visual arts' ability to utilise a specific kind of symbolism and metaphor, which work in a different way to narrative, with images or sculptures having a more direct and immediate impact on our consciousness and senses (Freeland 2010, pp. 189).

Aging can also be an important factor in body-dissatisfaction (Grogan, 2008 p.4; Cash & Szymanski, 1995). Hogan and Warren (2012) suggest that for women 'experiences of ageing are profoundly rooted in appearance' (p.329). Aging can make women feel 'invisible' (Skaife & Huet 1998, p.9; Thone 1992, p.79), as can being considered overweight or obese (Pausé 2007). Skaife & Huet (1998) suggest that art therapy offers older women an opportunity for self-expression and that it is important for art therapists to recognise and support the needs of this sector of our society (p.9). Working with older women can offer young art therapists a greater understanding of the issues and needs that older women face. However, it is important to recognise the potential for a double transference when a young therapist works with older women (ibid.). In her art therapy research using clay with older women, Abramowitz (2013) found that the clay image provided access to memories for the client (p.5), and suggested that the unique medium of clay created a positive – even a pleasurable – experience for the maker (p.4). For Abramowitz the self-directed and unstructured use of clay benefitted her older research participants, writing of a woman who destroyed then rebuilt her clay sculpture, allowing for self-expression and giving the client a voice (p.5).

The idea of 'visible mending' (Jones 2008; Carr 2015) is an important process and philosophy to consider when undertaking clay work with clients exploring body image, as it acknowledges both *imperfection* and *adaption* at the same time. Born out of the Japanese art of Kintsugi (金継ぎ) 'golden joinery' (also known as Kintsukuroi [金繕い] or 'golden repair'), it is a process used in ceramics, where cracked or broken areas are visibly repaired with seams of precious metal. The Ashmolean Museum in Oxford has on display an example of Kintsugi, where, instead of discarding or trying to invisibly mend a broken tea bowl, the cracks have been lovingly overlaid in gold, so as to accentuate the 'visible mending', therefore the imperfections are celebrated markers of authenticity, giving the bowl additional worth.

The Japanese values of Wabi-Sabi (a philosophy of aesthetics) underpin this tradition and translate as 'All things are impermanent; All things are imperfect; All things are incomplete; "Greatness" exists in the inconspicuous and overlooked details; and beauty can be coaxed out of ugliness' (Koren, 1998, pp.46–51). Wabi-Sabi is also an appreciation of that which is unpretentious or irregular; it is the finding of beauty in imperfection, which reminds us of the transient nature of life, yet celebrates the natural cycle of growth and decay and finally death.

Media and Cultural Influence on Body Image

The body in Western society has been 'informed and inscribed' by social, political and cultural discourses, and influenced by other disciplines, such as aspects of sociology and philosophy (Cancienne & Snowber 2009, p.199). Feminist researchers have historically viewed women as victims within a society that attempts to control them through their bodies (Grogan 2008, p.75). In the 1980s, a series of unrealistic ideals and expectations or 'beauty norms' for women around body image, were identified (e.g. women expected to be slender but with large breasts), meaning it was impossible for most women to meet these ideals (ibid.). When the media promote unrealistic cultural body image representations, women are left feeling unattractive and unlovable, and end up in a state of disembodiment, rejecting and attempting to change or control their bodies.

The Institute for the Psychology of Eating (https://psychologyofeating.com/connections-body-image-shame/) claim that during any given day – on average – 97% of women say that they dislike or are ashamed of their own bodies, and the main source of shame for women is their weight. Some of the ways that we attempt to control our bodies/weight is through harmful activities, such as cosmetic surgery, depriving ourselves of food, and often joyless exercise. With regards dieting people often berate themselves if they do not achieve their goals, labeling this as a 'lack of will power' – something that causes further feelings of shame – and the vicious cycle continues.

Problematised Bodies and Gender

According to objectification theory (Frederickson & Roberts, 1997), women's bodies have also, over centuries, been socially constructed as 'objects', that can be looked at and judged (Grogan 2008, p.74). Girls learn that to gain social approval, they must continually evaluate themselves against the current trends in body image (Grogan 2008, p.74). This continual self-evaluation can therefore lead to feelings of body-shame when they do not fit into the current norm (Grogan 2008, p.75). Particularly where a person has been treated as an 'object', as in physical abuse, shame can be particularly devastating, as it often occurs in a context where unconditional love and care or 'special personal recognition is expected', e.g. between a parent and child, or within other emotional and sexual relationships (Fonagy et al. 2003, p.445).

As soon as a child is born, they and their bodies are ascribed cultural meanings purely on the basis of what sex they are, and while it is impossible to escape cultural influence entirely, it is important to question the process of normalisation around gender that happens within socially constructed institutions (Hogan 2003 p.14). As Butler (2006 p.26) says:

> Constituted as a social phenomenon in the public sphere, my body is and is not mine. Given over from the start to the world of others, it bears their imprint, is formed within the crucible of social life; only later, and with some uncertainty, do I lay claim to my body as my own, if, in fact, I ever do.

As therapists it is important to understand and challenge the cultural constructions around gender, so that we can avoid imposing 'preconceived or universalised' ideas on our clients, about what constitute 'gender norms' in therapy (Hogan 2003, p.21). It is important therefore to understand the key role that cultural and social representations of gender play in how people see themselves (Hogan 2003, p.12), and understand how the impact of gender stereotypes affects the way people are treated within society and the lack of opportunities or limits that are placed on them (Hogan 1997).

Clearly 'body-image is a multidimensional phenomenon' (Cash & Pruzinsky 2002b, p.7), and arguably women experience objectification of their bodies and genders from multiple different sources and, at least in developed countries, the message has historically been that the female body is something to be 'looked at, evaluated, possessed by men, and, in general, treated as an object' (Levine & Smolak 2002, p.81). There has also been a tendency to link the physical attractiveness of a person with positive qualities, with Dion and colleagues coining the phrase 'What is beautiful is good' (Dion et al. 1972, p.285).

Research has shown that for most people, it is their friends, family and social media, that provide the relevant social information about acceptable or unacceptable body image, which highlights the importance of researching body image within its specific cultural context (Grogan 2008), e.g. mother–daughter relationships. Generally, women also score lower than men in evaluations of appearance satisfaction, and higher on preoccupations with weight, with the areas of the body that cause most concern for women being the stomach, buttocks and hips (Cath et al. 1986; Grogan 2008; Striegel-Moore & Franko 2002).

Not fitting into positive cultural body image norms, means that people can face prejudice throughout their lives, with overweight people being treated differently from childhood (Cash 1990). Children learn about body image norms early on, they tend to play less with their overweight peers, and are able to assign negative words to drawings of obese people (ibid.). This learned prejudice is often carried into adulthood, with overweight people discriminated against, e.g. when renting property, applying for jobs or college places etc. (ibid.). Being overweight for both males and females, is also generally considered physically unattractive, although this has not always been the case, with larger fleshy women particularly characterised as 'beautiful' by Renaissance artists such as Peter Paul Rubens [1577–1640].

Religious influences may also have historically and even today played their part, with gluttony and greed two of the seven deadly sins outlined to early Christians by Pope Gregory the First, in approximately the year 600 (https://www.bibleinfo.com/en/questions/what-are-seven-deadly-sins). Western societies, therefore, consider slenderness as socially acceptable and it is associated with success, happiness, and youthfulness, whereas obesity is linked to lack of willpower, laziness, and lack of control (Grogan 2008, p.9).

From a medical perspective the consequences of obesity have been well-researched and documented; however, the psychological effects are less clear (Schwartz & Brownell 2002 p.200). It is generally assumed that people who are overweight or obese will have a poor body image and feel ashamed of their bodies; however this assumption is a reflection of the powerful social stigma against them (ibid.), with research revealing a more complex picture. Indeed, some people have a more positive view of their bodies despite being overweight or obese, and for those who have a poor body image some people are severely affected and some less so, and a poor body image does not necessarily decrease with weight loss (ibid.).

It seems clear therefore that body image is subjective, often bearing no correlation between what is perceived by an outside observer and a person's subjective experience of their own bodies (Grogan 2008, p.4). In Chapter 3 we discuss the neurological implications behind this discrepancy, something that is particularly apparent in people diagnosed with eating disorders, especially anorexia nervosa. However, this phenomenon is not just evident in extreme cases, as women/girls who are considered average or below average in a weight/height ratio, often report feeling 'fat' (ibid.).

A behavioural indicator of a poor body image is the continued attempts to change one's body shape and weight through diet, something that most women have attempted at some time in their lives, and something that is advocated by many women's magazines (Grogan, 2008 pp.57–58), television and social media. Recent studies have confirmed that eating disorders are prevalent worldwide, particularly among women (Galmiche et al. 2019). Whilst we acknowledge that body image issues and eating disorders affect men as well as women (Delderfield 2018), this book, and the study from which the case studies are drawn, focused only on women.

Not only is a poor body image a psychiatric condition, it can also be deadly, with the mortality rate in the USA for people diagnosed with anorexia nervosa being higher than that of any other psychiatric condition, and is approximately 10x higher than that of the general population (Birmingham & Treasure 2010, p.1; Battaglia & McNamara 2012, p. 50). This highlights the seriousness of body image issues, particularly those that include eating disorders as a coping mechanism. An unhealthy focus given to 'beauty' and idealised bodies in the media, means that many women are denied positive reflections of themselves, from very early in life to older age (Ellis 1989, p.119).

There is a tension between images of idealised 'fit' bodies in the media, which may encourage people to lose weight, eat healthily, take more exercise, and the effect these images may have on people who are overweight, perhaps 'giving up' and feeling unable to partake in sport or exercise because their bodies don't fit in to that culture (Grogan 2008, p.5). Also, a positive body image may be an influencing factor in whether people eat healthily or whether they binge eat or restrict their eating, with a positive body image meaning they are less likely to engage in self-destructive behaviours around food (ibid.). It is not surprising therefore that a positive body image is associated with high self-esteem (ibid. p.44).

It has been assumed by researchers that older women have body shape ideals similar to those of younger groups, influenced by advertising in the media of body shape ideals (Ussher 1993), however it has been argued that older people have a more realistic, age-related, heavier ideal body size (Lamb et al. 1993), suggesting that people may adjust their ideal body shape as they get older and gain extra weight (Grogan 2008, p.154). However, other studies have shown that body dissatisfaction in women does not change with age until they are quite elderly (Grogan 2008).

Many women believe, due to the normative beliefs around the idealisation of ultra-slim bodies in the media, that they must look a certain way to fit in or be acceptable to society, and this results in a belief they should be able to *control* the size and fitness of their bodies. A failure to do so can result in feelings of guilt and depression, and judgements from society that they are lazy, lacking in willpower, greedy, and even amoral.

The female body continues to be objectified and problematised, with a continual drive from advertising and social media, to 'improve' one's health and body image, something that feeds the need for consumers to buy new products (Evans 2005, pp.44–45). This leads to a belief that by changing our bodies or external props (e.g., weight, clothes, hair colour, breast size, nose etc.), we can make ourselves more acceptable within society, relationships and even improve our relationship with ourselves (ibid.). This encourages a distorted relationship with our bodies, with – on the one hand – the 'perfect' body set on a pedestal and idealised, and on the other a body that becomes a focus for depression, anxiety and self-hatred, characterised by anorexia nervosa and obesity, the two extremes of eating disorders (ibid. p.43).

Attachment Theory, Body Image, and the Mother–Daughter Relationship

If body image is built through relationships, the earliest key relationship is generally that created with the baby and its earliest carers. For the purpose of this book we focus on the mother–daughter relationship, although we acknowledge that other early relationships, such as that between father and daughter etc may be equally important. In order to explore these early relationships, it is important to develop an understanding of attachment theory, and to explore how these theories support the idea of using clay work as an intervention for exploring body image issues in women, and indeed the possibility of inheriting or learning body image issues from their mothers and grandmothers, as well as from culture and social media.

Kenneth Wright's (2009) theory of 'mirroring and attunement' develops and connects Donald Winnicott's (1971b) ideas about mother/baby *mirroring*, with Daniel Stern's (1985) thesis on *attunement.* Stern's thesis (1985) describes the complex process where a mother reflects her baby's affective states back to the baby, as a way to promote self-awareness and validate the baby's experience, whilst also *attuning* their response in a way that attempts to change that experience, e.g., by exaggerating surprise or downplaying distress. Whilst Stern's research was mainly concerned with the early mother–baby relationship, he also believed that attunement is important *throughout a person's life* (1985 p.23). Wright builds on the ideas of art critic Peter Fuller (1980) to argue that the surfaces of an artwork (e.g., the clay sculptures featured in this book), function as a 'responsive and mirroring extension of the self' or as a 'surrogate adaptive mother' (Wright 2009, p.13).

Studies have shown that a positive 'good enough (m)other'–baby relationship is crucial to a child's normal development (Winnicott 1975, p.10; Wright 2009), however, what is less known is the way that a mother's view of herself and her body (both positive and negative views) influence the way baby girls view and experience their own bodies (Fuerstein 2009, p.21). Even in the womb the mother's voice and touch will send messages to her baby that begin to form the way her baby will see herself in later life (ibid.). (We have used the word (m)other (Wright 2009) with the bracketed 'm' to demonstrate our understanding that not all babies/children are brought up by their mothers; for some the 'mothering' is offered by 'others').

Research has shown that the mother–daughter relationship is a place where body image issues can be passed down from mother to daughter, grandmother to granddaughter and even great-grandmothers to great-granddaughters (Arroyo et. al. 2017, p.10); therefore parents who are anxious about their own looks and weight are, inadvertently, likely to pass these anxieties on to their children, and these can be historical issues passed down through the generations (ibid.). As Fuerstein (2009) says, '[. . .] if your mother has a distorted self-image, it's likely she'll view you through her own inaccurate lens – especially if she sees you and herself as one' (p.4). Also, Ernst (1987) and Orbach (1997) suggest that a mother's own unmet needs may unconsciously cause her to thwart her daughter's initiatives, and thus discourage her from being guided by her own intuition (Waldman 1999, p.11).

In order to really *know* her baby, an attuned mother must be able to *see* her baby, not as an extension of the self – with all her own distorted beliefs about her body image defects, but as a new individual (Fuerstein 2009, p.21). The word 'see' is also not just a reference to the visual nature of 'seeing', but also means for a mother to recognise her daughter as a unique individual, with personal likes, dislikes and dreams that should, if possible, be respected (ibid. p.198). Sharing a common gender means there is often an intensified bond which increases the impact of the mother's gaze on her daughter, and it is necessary to form a strong attachment before the mother gradually separates from her, allowing a more objective view of one's self to form (ibid.). A mother's negative attitude towards her daughter's body may also get magnified by the daughter for survival reasons, as her life or death depends upon this relationship being positively maintained (ibid. p.21)

For babies and toddlers, the body is the main way of communicating with their mother, the body also 'keeps the score' of how the infant is treated by the mother. As Wallin (2007) says, 'the [infant] body remembers as well as reveals' (p.293). It seems that our earliest primal body-mind experiences are 'encoded' in the brain's memory, and can be reawakened later in life, when situations similar to those experienced with caregivers happen (Fuerstein 2009, p.83).

Fuerstein describes the process of successfully managing an infant's distress as the 'hug cycle' (Fuerstein 2009, p.83). She also describes an unsuccessful attachment as the 'carnival mirror' which is 'a mirror which offers back, not a true reflection of who you are, but a *distorted* image' (ibid. p.2). For the purposes of this book, we choose to call this the 'distorted mirror' – as the word 'carnival' indicates something fun and pleasurable. The term 'distorted mirror' describes how a mother who has not sufficiently detached from her daughter, is unable to see her as an independent being, and therefore unconsciously views her daughter through her own distorted lens and influences the daughter's view of herself in a negative (and most probably false) way. Therefore, a mother who has an inaccurate view of herself, can pass on this inaccurate self-view to her daughter (Fuerstein 2009, p.16).

Some mothers – especially those with a distorted self-image – also tend to overlook their daughters because they are preoccupied with their own worries and have difficulty seeing their daughters as individuals (Fuerstein 2009, p.65). It is also likely that these mothers experienced a similar relationship with *their* mothers, they are therefore unconsciously perpetuating an historical negative relationship trait (ibid. p.66). Daughters in such relationships, who experience a distorted self-image, can often feel that part of their self-worth comes from acting as a 'special helper' or developing a 'make it better' role with their mothers (Fuerstein 2009, p.17). This often requires the daughters to give up their own needs in order to support their mothers and to feel accepted. This 'barter system' means that, in order to feel accepted, daughters are often required to 'yield control' to their mother (Fuerstein 2009, p.120). In a child's mind, if you can't be loved (or are made to feel unlovable), then at least *be needed*, which may at least ensure the child's long-term survival. After all, the helplessness of a baby or child can mean that the mother is seen as significantly more large and powerful, her anger more scary and her lack of empathy or care more unacceptable (Fuerstein 2009, p.37).

For a healthy mother–daughter relationship, the daughter must feel nurtured by the mother, but also feel empowered to return that nurturing to their mother (Stern 1985). This is a healthy mirroring, that builds a positive sense of self-worth. However, mothers that are unable to 'see' their daughters, are unable to show that they are affected by them (Fuerstein 2009 p.197). When preoccupied mothers look at their daughters, they often see a reflection of themselves, this can even be true of mothers who are less self-absorbed, due to sharing a common gender (Fuerstein 2009, p.198). Daughters of preoccupied mothers can learn that their individuality must be supressed, as love and attention is dependent upon being like their mothers (ibid.). For Winnicott (1960, pp.140–157), this results in what he called 'the false self', where the expectations of other people can override or contradict a person's original sense of self, and such children may also go on to develop a poor body image.

Fuerstein (2009, p.53) describes the *hug cycle* as the process of soothing carried out instinctively by the good enough (m)other, which leads to a *sense of security* in the infant, and results in the infant going from a place of frustration and rage to feeling comforted and soothed. The sense of security this gives the infant is important, as neuroscientists claim that this helps to develop the child's 'social brain', which are areas of the non-verbal brain that are shaped by early relationships (Cozolino 2006). A sense of security is developed when (m)others use the hug cycle and tune in to their baby's needs to help them cope with discomfort. On the other hand, if (m)others are tuned out from their baby, with inward-looking traits, then the baby will experience the opposite of the hug cycle, something Fuerstein calls the '*boomerang cycle*' (Fuerstein 2009, p.53). The '*boomerang cycle*' is where the (m)other is so focused on her own needs that she is unable to tune into her baby's needs, which leads to the baby displaying 'frustration, rage, lack of comforting, more rage – the boomerang cycle, which leads to insecurity' (ibid. p.54).

Puberty can be a time when girls in particular struggle with a more negative body image, due to a natural increase in weight and body mass, which can lead to a preoccupation with dieting and fitness; also existing issues may be accentuated during puberty (Levine & Smolak 2002, p.75). Children and adolescents may also experience peer and family teasing about their bodies, something that has been shown to be implicated in adult body issues. However, it has also been argued that people who experience poor body image may be more likely to recall and report experiences such as being teased as a child (Schwartz & Brownell 2002, p.206).

For girls, early adolescence is a particularly important period in the development of body image, as a positive or negative body image is influential in normative development in sexuality, self-identity formation, gender role development, and exploring a range of realistic possibilities in important areas of their lives (Levine & Smolak 2002, p.75). One reason that girls in particular are prone to preoccupations about their weight and body image, is because – as they go through puberty and adolescence – it has been found that parents are more likely to offer their daughters criticism, rather than praise, for their appearance (ibid. p.80).

The impact of a negative body image is often felt throughout a person's life. As children we are like sponges, soaking up everything we hear said about us, and these things are taken as the 'truth', meaning that as adults we are unable to believe positive statements that contradict these early learned 'truths' (Fuerstein 2009, p.2). As women approach and live through the menopause, body image issues may be exacerbated; however, if her childhood experiences were more of the 'hug cycle,' as opposed to the 'boomerang cycle', and these were continued throughout her life, it stands to reason that she will be more resilient to the onslaught of the menopause (Fuerstein 2009, p.95). Equally, if she experienced more of the 'boomerang cycle' growing up, signs of aging will bring back feelings of body image dissatisfaction and discomfort (ibid.).

Positive body image experiences from childhood are also remembered throughout life. Barbara Marcus (2004) describes a middle-aged patient who talks of her own positive body image experiences with her mother, that have sustained her into old age, saying:

> 'She'd put her large, square hands in mine and say mine were lovely, so artistic, so soft and white. She'd worked in factories all her life . . . I still love my hands, in spite of arthritis and age spots. [. . .] Isn't it odd that mother's appreciation in the end is still what makes them lovely to me?'
>
> (patient quoted in Marcus 2004, p.88)

It seems clear therefore that daughters often model themselves on their mothers' negative or positive beliefs about their own body image (Choate 2015, p.1; Jaffe & Worobey 2006, p.3), and negative beliefs correlate with the daughters experiencing increased body image issues and eating disorders (Cooley et al. 2008). On the other hand, studies have shown that a mother's positive emotional support correlates with an increase in a daughter's positive body image (Shenaar-Golan & Walter 2015, p.555). The risk of developing eating disorders is also linked to the attachment styles experienced as a child, with those experiencing insufficient care and high levels of control much more likely to develop eating disorders (Battaglia & McNamara 2012; Swanson et al. 2009).

Attachment Theory, Body-Shame, and 'Covering Up'

Within attachment theory 'emotional sharing and signaling' are the primary mechanisms for the regulation of attachment security (Herman 2018, p.158). Infants develop self-consciousness in their second year, when they react to their caregivers' emotional signals, to learn what others think of them, and what is acceptable and what isn't, generally reacting with shame when approval is withheld or withdrawn (ibid.). The sharp pain of shame associated with failure to please their (m)other causes the child to fear the loss of relationship and brings with it associated feelings of hopelessness or isolation (Trevarthen 2005). However, within a secure attachment, the child learns that feelings of shame can be overcome and only result in a temporary suspension of emotional attunement with their care givers (Herman 2018, p.158).

In a study by Daye et al. (2014), examining the link between restrictive or critical caregiver eating messages and body-shame/self-compassion, it was found that in a sample of 322 U.S. college women, there was a strong link between negative and critical eating messages from caregivers and the participant's experiences of body-shame (p.547). The study also found that those experiencing body-shame were less able to mitigate feelings of shame through self-compassion (ibid.). Body-shame can also extend beyond body size and shape, is often distorted and negative, and can leave people feeling 'unworthy' of pleasure and play. When a person feels 'ashamed', this speaks of an inter-personal experience, where the person shamed recognises themselves as 'a - *shamed*' person.

One of the themes immediately evident within the data from Session One was that of 'covering up', either metaphorically or physically, those body parts that the participants were anxious about showing. This 'covering up' indicated that these were parts of their bodies that engendered feelings of shame. Shame is the feeling of being *flawed* and needing to be *fixed* in order to be accepted and loved; also body-shame usually involves comparing one's body to others, and as such is generally about competition and conformity (Brown 2006, p.16).

Shame and Guilt

Shame and guilt are often referred to as 'moral emotions' (Shen 2018, p.1), mediated by moral and social beliefs or 'norms.' Shame and guilt are both painful and negative emotions, but they have important differences that can be overlooked (Tangney et al. 2006). Shame can be described as 'the imagined critical perception of others' to one's self or actions, whereas guilt results from one's own critical judgement, judging one's self or one's actions (Pulcu et al. 2014, p.1). Shame means 'I am the problem' and someone else knows it, whereas guilt means 'I recognise that I did something wrong' and no one else necessarily knows about it. Feelings of shame may bring about behaviours such as attempting to hide or deny the object of shame, whilst feelings of guilt may bring about behaviours such as attempting to amend or compensate for any wrongdoing (Tangney et al. 2006).

Sznycer et al. (2016) claim that shame is an important evolutionary and adaptive emotion, in that it defends against social devaluation, by ensuring people avoid showing that which would result in more devaluation than benefits, with their data showing a correlation between the intensity of shame felt and the amount of perceived personal social devaluation (p.2625).

The social expressions of shame, e.g., lowered eyes, bowed head and hiding one's self, are also signals of a subordinate social status (Herman

2018, p.163). The emotions associated with shame include 'shyness, self-consciousness, embarrassment, and feeling foolish or ridiculous', and it is through these experiences that the boundaries around what behaviour is socially acceptable, are learned (ibid. p.162). Extreme reactions to shame may result from being treated in a degrading manner, and include 'humiliation, self-loathing, and feelings of defilement, disgrace, or dishonour' (ibid.). This can cause a cumulative reaction as people diagnosed with major depressive disorder (MDD) are particularly prone to self-blame emotions such as guilt and shame, and may indicate a vulnerability even after recovery (Pulcu et al. 2014, p.1).

Shame, Resilience, and Self-Compassion

Self-compassion can be described as having three elements, i.e. self-kindness, common human experience and mindfulness (Neff 2003; Brown 2006). Self-kindness is the ability to be nurturing and understanding to ourselves instead of self-critical when we experience failure, suffering or feelings of inadequacy. Common human experience recognises that feelings of foolishness, inferiority, and suffering are things that all human beings experience. Mindfulness is about facing negative emotions and recognising them without exaggerating or over-identifying with them, so as to ensure a sense of balance and self-compassion (Neff 2003; Brown 2006).

The role of self-compassion as an antidote to body-shame has been highlighted in a number of recent studies (Daye et al. 2014; Ferreira et al. 2013; McBeth & Gumley, 2012), with Ferreira et al. (2013) discovering that a reduced ability for self-compassion was linked to 'a stronger experience of the self as living negatively in the mind of others, with increased general psychopathology and disordered eating symptomatology' (p.207). Their findings also indicate a general drive for thinness in women (from the general population), who experienced feelings of shame associated with body image (ibid.). However, self-compassion in the face of body-shame and dissatisfaction has been found to correlate with a positive body image, and consequently reduced body modifying behaviours such as eating disorders (Ferreira et al. 2013, p.207). This highlights the growing empirical evidence regarding the importance of developing self-compassion in women as a strategy for emotional regulation, particularly for those who experience body image dissatisfaction and feelings of body-shame (Ferreira et al. 2013; McBeth & Gumley, 2012).

Shame is one of the most universal and primitive of human emotions, and although shame is under-researched, studies have begun to explore the strategies women use in order to develop 'shame resilience' (Brown 2006, p.43). Brown (2006) discovered the importance of women finding their voice regarding shame, something she identified as the importance of 'speaking shame', which can be facilitated within psychoeducational group work, as well as the development of empathic relationships and the acknowledgement of vulnerability (p.43). Therefore, it seems that shame doesn't survive being spoken about and being met with empathy, self-compassion, and understanding; instead shame thrives on silence, secrecy, and judgement (by the self or others) (Brown 2006).

Aging and Body Image

Given that 'beauty' and the 'perfect body' are seen in Western Society as the domain of the young and slim, older women face enormous challenges in their efforts to develop and preserve a positive body image (Hurd 2000, p.77) and self-identity (Carr 2018). This is not helped by a lack of research and publication on body image for older women, meaning that many of the complex issues older women face have been largely ignored (Kilpela et al. 2015, p.144; Ferraro et al. 2008). In contrast there is a plethora of literature investigating body image issues experienced by young adult women and adolescents (Kilpela et al. 2015).

The issue of poor body image in older women was highlighted in a study carried out in 2006 by Mangweth-Matzek et al., whereby 500 women (aged 60–70 years) were questioned about their body image and eating habits. The results demonstrated that over 60% of women reported body dissatisfaction, and 56% described restricting their food intake as a way to prevent weight gain (ibid.). In a further study it was found that the percentage of body image dissatisfaction did not differ between younger and older women (Bedford & Johnson 2006), which seems to indicate that women experience body image dissatisfaction throughout their lifetime (Ferraro et al. 2008). One difference may be that older women are less influenced by pressure to conform to media ideals than younger women (Lewis & Cachelin 2001; Ferraro et al. 2008).

It seems clear that older women have body image issues that differ from and are more complex than those of younger women, as aging brings with it physiological age-related changes, the menopause, the effects of medication, and other issues related to psychological changes and altered priorities in lifestyle (Kilpela et al. 2015, p.144). Physiological age-related changes include a general reduction in muscle mass and an increase in fat mass; there is also a redistribution of fat from the legs and buttocks to the stomach and abdomen, as well as changes to the hair, skin tone, and elasticity (Tchkonia et al. 2010). Psychological and emotional issues may also be more prevalent due to the loss of a parent or partner. However, data has also suggested that the anxiety over body image lessens with age (Tiggemann & Lynch 2001), as does a preoccupation with thinness (Lewis & Cachelin 2001). Further to this, as people approach advanced age, there is often a growing tension between a preoccupation with bodily appearance or bodily function (Cameron et al. 2019; Roy & Payette 2012).

Perhaps the most important thing to acknowledge is that women still care about their appearance despite advancing age and may use cosmetics, or other interventions, in order to appear as young as possible (Gosselink et al. 2008). This behaviour may also be influenced by the social stigma of aging, and the propensity for age to bring about feelings of invisibility, particularly for women

(Hurd & Griffin 2008). Feeling invisible is a painful experience, as it means no longer being seen for who you are, and no longer feeling validated by or worthwhile to the wider community. Unfortunately, as long as appearance is used as a measure of a woman's value, older women will be stigmatised and the pressure to 'age gracefully' will be to look *young* for as long as possible.

Body image issues for women in later life may also be influenced by society norms, the media, and also by a lifetime of experiences (both positive and negative), from childhood, puberty, young adulthood, and middle age. Many complex factors will therefore influence how older women experience their bodies, and the participants in this study explored these through the unique properties of clay work, in order to understand where these views originated from, and how they can adapt, change, or accept them.

Within this chapter we have explored attachment theory and the development of body image, with particular reference to mirroring and attunement and the mother–daughter relationship. Research was discussed that indicates a strong link between mothers' and daughters' body image issues, suggesting that daughters see themselves through a *distorted mirror* – that of their mother's own distorted body image. The importance of building self-compassion and resilience was also highlighted, as a way to counter feelings of guilt and shame. Other influential factors such as aging and gender were also explored as a theoretical background to the case study phenomenological analysis, which will be discussed in Chapter 6.

3 Making Connections

Metaphor, Evolution, and Neuroscience

Metaphor and Embodied Cognition

Human beings enjoy using metaphors, often using them many times a day, meaning that they are so ingrained in everyday conversation that they are often spoken without noticing (Lai et al. 2019). The importance of metaphor and symbolism within this study has been the belief that metaphorical language and thought, and our capacity to understand it, is 'grounded in embodiment' (Gibbs, Costa & Francozo 2004, p.1189).

The use of metaphor in linguistics is increasingly being viewed as a central component of higher cognition and abstract thought (Coulson & Lai 2016). Most research into what happens in the brain when we think metaphorically vs literally, has been concerned with discovering a relationship between the two (Coulson & Lai 2016). Lakoff suggests that a 'cascade' of diverse brain circuitry is required when handling metaphoric language or abstract thought, 'linking many diverse brain regions to allow for the indefinitely large variety of human reason and imagination' (Lakoff 2014 p.12).

Cognitive neuroscience therefore suggests that our 'cognition' or ability to reason, is grounded in our bodily experiences or embodiment, something that Lakoff calls 'embodied cognition' (Lakoff 2014, p.2). This is in sharp contrast to René Descartes' 17th-century theory of 'dualism' or the mind–body divide, whereby he claimed that the mind or soul of man is entirely different and distinct from the body (Descartes 1996 [1641], p.136.). Lakoff (2014) explains that embodiment makes concepts meaningful, enabling the linking of what is going on in our brains to an understanding of what is going on in the real world. Lakoff also suggests that for abstract concepts to be understood they have to be given embodied meaning, therefore 'embodied metaphor is a major mechanism for characterizing how we understand abstract concepts' (Lakoff 2014, p.7). This highlights embodiment as a central mechanism of meaningfulness, and therefore the importance of embodied metaphors within clay work and body image.

Metaphors enable us to employ familiar, concrete domains, to rationalise abstract concepts, that can then be applied flexibly to understand new issues and situations (Jamrozik et al. 2016, p.1080). Studies have also shown that sentences which employ metaphor are more emotionally engaging than those that contain literal content (Citron & Goldberg 2014). Also, the use of metaphor may prompt a form of embodied simulation, e.g. within descriptions of pain where the words 'burning' or 'stabbing', may elicit an empathic response (Samino 2010, p.205).

Metaphor and symbolism were used intuitively by many of the women who took part in this study, often employing a process of imaginative thinking to add meaning and significance to their sculptures. Neuroaestheticists Ramachandran & Hirstein (1999) discovered that metaphor is an important aspect of the aesthetic appreciation in art, and provide a useful description of metaphor for this study as 'a mental tunnel between two concepts or precepts that appear grossly dissimilar on the surface' (p.31).

The ability to share and understand metaphor and symbolism within the therapeutic relationship is a vitally important factor within art therapy and clay work, and equates to being, or feeling 'in touch' with another person. This requires that each understands the other's 'symbolic capability', and it is this mutual understanding that enables metaphor or symbolism to be recognised, and learned from within the work (Wright 2009, p.25).

Visual art utilises a specific kind of symbolism and metaphor, both of which work in a different way to narrative, containing a symbolism that goes beyond the surface (Dissanayake 1995, p.20). The incorporation of metaphor and symbolism is also a key way that self-images – be they painted or sculpted in clay – are able to hold dualities such as hope and despair (Clayton et al. 2005, 2008; Carr 2015).

Images are special, as they can have a direct and immediate impact on our consciousness (Freeland 2010; Kramer 2004), whereas metaphor and symbolism work in a more subtle way, and require the creator and the viewer to be on the same level of understanding. The ability of metaphor and symbolism to hold and represent ambiguity and tacit knowledge is an important factor in how they work (Hatch & Yanow 2008). Tacit knowledge is knowledge that cannot be verbalised and therefore can only become known when it is 'expressed through symbolic forms' (Jongeward 2009, p.241) such as artworks, where ambiguity is possible and interpretation is often fluid and adaptable (Carr 2015, p.50). After all,

> [a]rt by its very nature has the deviant potential for ambiguity. It has the capacity for holding many notions, many angles, many colours and places, in a way that the written or spoken word rarely allows.
>
> (Jones 2003, p. 98)

One of the important functions of the therapist within art therapy, is their capacity to *hold*, metaphorically, the affect or experiences brought to the session by the client. The artworks created around those experiences also hold these experiences, but they are separated from the client and can therefore be looked at as separate. Within a phenomenological study, metaphor and symbolism can also be seen as another way to reduce complex phenomena to their *essence*.

Humour was used by many of the women taking part in the study, with laughter often punctuating their narrative. Humour utilises complex forms of metaphor and symbolism within the language used, with double innuendos and satire requiring an intricate understanding of context and social meaning. Humour can be used to 'lighten the atmosphere' in difficult situations, and to demonstrate feelings of appreciation and gratitude, to others (Weisfeld 1993). It is sometimes described as a 'ludic' defence mechanism or 'black humour' (Turner 1982, p.27), and can help people face and manage embarrassment, trauma, and liminality, and relieve tension. As Brown (2010, p.262) says:

> Laughter, song, and dance create emotional and spiritual connection; they remind us of the one thing that truly matters when we are searching for comfort, celebration, inspiration, or healing: We are not alone. Shame resilience requires laughter.

Humour is also an *imaginative way of being* (Hellema 2011), within which a sense of intimacy and connection can be created, through the tacit intersubjective knowing required to understand personalised humour. It is a way of testing the intersubjective connection and empathy by metaphorically asking "Do you get it? Do you get me?" and also "Do you *know* me?" (Carr 2015, p.124). Brown (2010, p.263) refers to this as 'knowing laughter', something that embodied the feelings of 'relief and connection we experience when we realize the power of sharing our stories—we're not laughing at each other but with each other' (ibid.). Research has shown that more laughter and less embarrassment occur when people of equal status are present (Fink & Walker, 1977), therefore the humour expressed by the participants may indicate that they recognised the similarities between each other and felt comfortable within the group.

Humour can be seen as intrinsically 'adaptive' (Carr 2018, p.128), it can help with developing a sense of perspective and managing stressful situations, and can create a sense of *emotional distance* (Hellema 2011, p.163). However, it is important when working with clients to ensure that humour is initially client-led, to ensure that the art therapist is aware of the limits and boundaries of the client's humour.

Metaphor and symbolism are often used in rituals, and both art and rituals are 'bracketed', or set apart from the mundane and ordinary. Ritual and symbolism within art therapy processes are particularly valuable in 'metaphorizing the body' (Sibbett 2005, pp.71–72), enabling the expression of 'emotions and bodily states including conscious and unconscious aspects otherwise deemed unspeakable, unbearable, unseeable and unthinkable' (ibid.).

Creating art is often a process of merging the 'sensory/sensuous experience of storytelling with the sensory/sensuous immediacy of visual representations' we find ourselves in an 'in between space' which is 'dialogic, visual' (O'Neill 2008, p.11), but also a *potential* or *interpsychic space* (Winnicott 1971a). This takes the artist to a similar place of 'liminality', a place where rites of passage can be played out, and where feelings of 'ambiguity, embodied experience, chaos, playing with multifocal symbols, expression and transition' are explored. (Sibbett 2005, p.68; Turner 1995 [1969] p.109).

The theory of liminality originated within a seminal work by van Gennep (1960) on rites of passage and Turner's later work on ritual around rites of passage events (Turner 1995 [1969]). Major transitional life events such as marriage, childbirth, and death cause change and uncertainty and as such provoke profound anxiety; therefore, rituals such as weddings, baptisms, and funerals have developed within societies to provide a supportive framework where containment and witnessing are offered (van Gennep 1960). Changes to body image are also part and parcel of growing up and aging, with birthday parties being ritualistic occasions to mark becoming a year older.

Neuroscience, Neuroaesthetics, and Body Image

Increasingly neuroscientific research is being used as a way to explain the effective processes within art therapy (e.g. King et al. 2019; Guseva 2018; Carr 2014; Hass-Cohen & Carr 2008; Franklin, M. 2010; Hass-Cohen & Clyde Findlay 2009; Gussie Klorer 2005; Lusebrink 2004; O'Brien 2004). Within this book we have therefore explored evidence from published neuroscientific and neuro-psychological research as an explanatory tool for the effectiveness of clay work. One of the main issues surrounding the use of neuroscience to explain the effectiveness of art therapy is that it forces us to cross intellectual borders and engage with a scientific language that is foreign to us. However, just as looking through two eyes instead of one enables depth of field perception, by 'seeing the world through the different lenses of art and science and by integrating these perspectives, [we] arrive at a deeper understanding of reality' (Leonard Shlain, quoted in Huang 2009, p.26).

Therefore, neuroscience may help us understand the most fundamental aspects of our work, positively influence art therapy practice, and help us to define our own professional identity.

Also, possessing a working knowledge of the processes and functions of the brain is important for therapists, as it enables a 'neurodevelopmentally informed approach' (Perry 2009) that can be used to develop tailored interventions for specific client groups. (For a detailed description of areas of the brain identified as important for art therapy, see Lusebrink 2004, and Hass-Cohen & Carr 2008).

As clay work involves sensory, visual, and tactile stimuli, we have researched neuroscientific explanations that explore the effect of visual and tactile perception on memories, emotion, agency, and adaptation, and also how stress and trauma (e.g. caused by a negative body image) may negatively impact upon vision and mood.

Body Image and Visual Disturbances

In the past two decades neuroscientific and neuro-psychological studies (e.g. Sinai et al. 1998; Adolphs, 2004; Stefanucci et al. 2009; Zadra & Clore 2011 [review]; Riener et al. 2011; Guardia et al. 2012) have explored the effect of *stress, trauma* and *emotion* on visual perception. This research suggests that instead of the human visual system reproducing an accurate version of reality, what we perceive is altered systematically (Zadra & Clore 2011), with both positive and negative emotion influencing visual perception and attention in different ways (Jolij & Meurs 2011; Bubl et al. 2010). This is important when considering the emotional impact of a negative body image, and the impact this has on how we view the world.

In a study by Guardia et al. (2012), it was found that when patients diagnosed with anorexia nervosa were asked to judge whether a doorway was sufficiently wide enough for themselves and another person to pass through, they overestimated their size, saying the door was not wide enough, when in reality, it was easily wide enough. Guardia et al. (2012) speculate that anorexic patients may overestimate the size of their body because an *updated* view of their thin body has not occurred within the central nervous system.

Whilst the case studies discussed within this book do not involve women diagnosed with a specific eating disorder, it is useful to consider the current research taking place within neuroscience for this client group. In a review of the research by Riva (2010), evidence from neuroscience and psychology is cited which begins to explain why an altered perception of body image occurs in eating disorders (ED). The explanations are based on evidence indicating that spatial experience requires the integration of two different reference frames, i.e., the *egocentric* frame (first-person sensory experience of the self) processed in the praecuneus area of the brain dealing with short-term spatial memory, and the *allocentric* frame, which is involved in observing the self in a situation via imagination and draws on long-term spatial memory from the hippocampus and medial temporal lobes. For these two frames to integrate their information it is necessary for an updated view of the body's dimensions and motor patterns to be stored in long-term memory. When this fails to happen, long-term memory is not updated with the first-person sensory experience and the person becomes locked into an older body image representation (Riva & Gaudio 2018). It is hypothesised that the initial disruption may be caused by stress, and neuroimaging has demonstrated an impairment to hippocampus functioning in people diagnosed with eating disorders (Gaudio et al. 2018).

The effect of stress and emotion on perception may begin to explain why people who have altered perceptions of themselves, literally *see themselves differently*. Studies have also shown that the 'locked in' image can remain even after the initial stressor is removed (Munsteadt et al. 1997). In a systematic review of resting-state functional-MRI studies, Gaudio et al. (2016) concluded that 'several brain regions could be involved in body image disturbances and may sustain an impaired integration between real and perceived internal/external state of one's own body in AN [anorexia nervosa] patients' (p. 582).

Studies in neuropsychology (Sinai, Ooi & He 1998; Stefanucci et al. 2009; Riener et al. 2011) have also shown that different emotional states influence *how the world is seen*, e.g. people in a sad or depressed mood may perceive a hill to be markedly steeper than it is in reality, with those in a happy or positive mood able to judge the steepness more accurately (Riener et al. 2011). Studies have also shown that emotion has an enhancing effect on memory, meaning emotional events will be remembered more vividly than neutral events (Holland & Kensinger 2010. *Review*).

Emotional affect, such as feelings of sadness or depression, have also been found to influence a person's spatial attention, which can be described as a focus on either the 'global' broader picture, or the 'local' narrow/detailed picture in a specific circumstance (Gasper & Clore 2002; Rowe et al. 2007). Negative affect, plus narrow attentional processing, correlates with amygdala activity, which seems to result in *vigilance* for negatively arousing stimuli (Anderson & Phelps 2001). Therefore, the way one sees the world, including ourselves, is influenced not only by that which we know, remember, and believe, but also by *how wide our focus is* (ibid.). Changing one's focus from the 'local' to the 'global' picture, enables a shift of attention from that which causes anxiety and negative feeling, to that which expands and creates possibilities; this is relevant to body image when a person 'sees' only the negative 'parts of the body' rather than their 'whole' body as a person.

Studies in neuroscience have demonstrated the adaptive 'plastic' properties of the human brain, including its ability to adapt to changes in: physiology, the environment, and experience (Pascual-Leone et al. 2005, p.377). This suggests the ongoing potential for interventions, such as clay work, to enable change and adaption within clients, as 'behaviour will lead to changes in brain circuitry, just as changes in brain circuitry will lead to behavioural modifications' (ibid., p.379).

Vision, Body Image, and Evolution

Studies have shown that although people are generally accurate at evaluating others, people tend to view themselves with an 'optimism bias' (Trivers 2002). However, this may be dependent upon the mental health of the person and having a positive body image. Optimism bias is where people compare themselves favourably against an average person similar to themselves, as the person they compare themselves against is viewed as less human and less individual than themselves (Shepperd et al. 2002). This may be an evolutionary development, to promote self-esteem and ensure ongoing self-care.

In a study, photographs of participants were manipulated to make them seem more attractive or less attractive, and participants were then asked to choose the photo that was the accurate representation of themselves; on average people chose the photograph that had been made 20% more attractive (Epley & Whitchurch 2008). Due to the competitive nature of the world and the concern that people have around their own perceived social status and reproductive fitness, they are unable to judge their own value correctly, and employ a process of *self-signaling* to demonstrate to themselves their own value (Bodner & Prelec 2020). *Self-signaling* can often involve *costly* activity, such as purchasing luxury goods, overcoming challenges, or making charitable donations, even in secret (Yarosh, 2019b).

The evolution of the brain and its preference for 'attractiveness' and 'beauty' can be attributed to their use as measures of fitness, health and reproductive ability, but also because they have been (throughout evolutionary history) difficult to fake (Yarosh 2019b, p.6). The features that signal physical and reproductive health are known as 'costly signals' (Millar 2009), i.e. youth, the absence of disease, and high levels of hormones that indicate fertility (Yarosh 2019b, p.7). Cultural symbols have also been added to the list of costly signals used to highlight reproductive fitness, e.g. expensive and decorative jewelry and clothes, luxury housing and possessions, etc., however these could also be considered fake costly signals, thereby deceiving others regarding reproductive health and ability (ibid. p.7).

Costly signals around health and fitness are also faked through altering appearance by applying makeup, something studies have shown makes it more difficult for the brain to recognise faces (Ueda & Koyama 2010). Using hair dye to cover grey hair, and cosmetics to smooth out skin tone, reduces the perceived age of women (Fesler et al. 2005; Russell et al. 2018). Wearing makeup has been shown in research studies to have important social benefits, such as an increase in perceptions of a person's 'attractiveness, competence, likeability and trustworthiness' (Etcoff et al. 2011).

Upholding the value of costly signals against fakery is an important evolutionary quality, and our brains have been hardwired with a lie detector to detect fakes and cheating, with the frontal lobe and amygdala predominantly involved in this process (Shermer 2004). Women are able to outperform men on lie detection, inferring that they have more to lose if they are unable to identify faked *costly signals* in potential mates (Fink & Matts 2007).

The use of fake costly signals around health and fertility has also been found to have economic consequences, with male restaurant-goers giving waitresses who wear makeup more tips, and of larger amounts, than to waitresses who didn't wear makeup (Guegen & Jacob 2011). Interestingly, the 'Lipstick Effect' (first described by cosmetics tycoon Leonard Lauder), suggests that lipstick sales increase during economic downturns, as women instinctively purchase more products to enhance their appearance when the environment is more competitive (Hill et al. 2012). These fake costly signals amount to telling or 'wearing' a lie, and studies have found that when telling a lie (even an unconscious one) the most effective way to convince others is to believe the lie yourself, and natural selection has ensured that humans possess a self-deception mechanism (Trivers 2002) to fulfil the purpose of self-deception regarding their own youth and fitness.

Youth underlies the majority of the characteristics of facial attractiveness that people look for when judging attractiveness (Tatarunaite et al. 2005), and older faces are judged as less attractive and less likeable (Ebner 2008), meaning that aging can cause a decline in confidence and self-esteem (Gupta & Gilchrest 2005). Judgements around age (including skin and body health) are also used to assess a person's status in the community, their attractiveness as a partner, and reproductive/child-bearing potential (Korthase & Trenholme 1982; Kwart et al. 2012). Assessments about age often overlap those of health when judging attractiveness, and the whiteness of the sclera (whites of the eyes), correlates strongly with perceptions of health, 'beauty', and youth (Russell et al. 2014).

The amount of oestrogen a woman produces is also an indicator as to their fertility and in a research study Law Smith et al. (2005) found that women with higher oestrogen levels were rated as more attractive by both men and other women; however, when women wore make-up, women with lower oestrogen levels literally 'made-up' for this deficit and appeared more attractive to men and women. The use of eye makeup specifically has been found to increase the perceived size of a woman's eyes (Jones et al. 2018) and provides the greatest increase in perceived attractiveness (Samson et al. 2010). Cula et al. (2010) found that observers looked at the eyes of women wearing eye makeup 40% longer than women wearing no eye makeup, and where women wear full facial makeup, observes will look at their eyes 80% longer. The wearing of lipstick was found to increase the time observers focus on women's lips by 26% (Jones et al. 2015).

Beauty, Body Image, and Evolution

As the well-known geneticist Dr Theodosius Dobzhansky wrote (1973), 'nothing in biology makes sense except in the light of evolution", and similarly it can be argued that 'nothing in beauty makes sense except in light of the brain' (Yarosh 2019a, p.8). Brain imaging techniques (e.g. functional magnetic resonance imaging (fMRI) and magnetoencephalography (MEG), etc.) have been used by neuroscientists to investigate the neural underpinnings of preferences for human bodies and faces (e.g. Martín-Loeches et al. 2014; Di Dio et al. 2011) (Cattaneo 2020). People from all cultures have similar areas of the brain that are dedicated to evaluating the attractiveness of others (Yarosh 2019a, p.1).

Clearly the human body has evolved in ways that are not just about function, but are also about being attractive to others, and much time and money is spent on improving physical appearance (Yarosh 2019a, p.1). All cultures throughout the world agree on who is and who is not attractive (Langlois et al. 2000), and in all cultures the people believed to be most attractive generally acquire more resources (Yarosh 2019a, p.1), and have more children, than those believed to be less attractive (Jokela 2009). This suggests that judgements regarding physical attractiveness are part of our evolutionary human genetics (Yarosh 2019a, p.2). Even babies as young as 6 months were found to gaze for longer at faces judged to be attractive, and spend less time looking at faces judged to be unattractive (Ramsey et al. 2004).

Men and women employ different strategies to appear attractive to others; however, the underlying biological reasons for these strategies are linked to a 'natural selection' pressure for reproductive and economic success (Yarosh 2019a, p.1). Evolutionally, evaluations of attractiveness provide important cues about a person's fitness and health, indicating the quality of their genes and ability to successfully bear and raise offspring, and the attractiveness of a person is the key predictor for people securing their preferred mate (Halberstadt 2007).

Humans and animals both show a preference for symmetrical bodies, as this is seen as a sign of physical and developmental health (Alam & Dover 2021). Even though some minor physical variations have no impact on function, they do impact dramatically on the person's perceived attractiveness (Jones et al. 2004). This may indicate why all cultures prefer average faces (Rubenstein et al. 2002), as average faces may be those most familiar, and therefore require the least cognitive capacity to interpret or recognise (Halberstadt, 2007).

Clearly attractiveness or 'beauty' is not just an evolutionary ideal used to attract a mate, but can also be part of our status or position in a hierarchy of attractiveness with our same-sex peers (Yarosh 2019a, p.1). This brings in a level of competition that is encouraged by Western media and advertising, and with good reason, as studies have shown that a woman whose male partner contributes not only good genes but also significant resources, will, on average, achieve more success than a woman with a partner who does not provide such support (Thornhill & Gangestad 2008). It is not surprising, therefore, that our brains have developed complex systems to assess accurately the characteristics that make up human attractiveness, e.g. health, age and child bearing potential (Yarosh 2019a, p.2). Therefore, our own personal attractiveness and our ability to detect attractiveness in others are evolutionary traits (ibid.). There is a clear body image implication to this conundrum, as, when people believe they are attractive to others, they also have a higher sense of self-esteem (ibid. p.1), and a higher self-esteem is associated with lower rates of body dissatisfaction (Mellor et al. 2010).

Self-Referential Memory, Aesthetics, Emotion, and Metaphor

Most people have a desire to be perceived as attractive, and much of the fine arts have historically depicted images of human beauty (Yarosh 2019a, p.1) in their vast museums and art galleries. The context within which an image or object or art is seen has been shown to considerably alter the aesthetic value and meaning that people attach to it (Kirk et al. 2009, p.1125). In a fMRI research project, Kirk et al. (2009) showed artwork to people in different contexts. The fMRI data they gathered demonstrated that the aesthetic rating participants gave to artwork was substantially higher for images viewed in a *gallery*, which indicates that 'aesthetic judgments are significantly biased by subjects' prior expectations about the likely hedonic value of stimuli according to their source' (Kirk et al. 2009, p.1125).

Aesthetic experiences have been termed the 'aesthetic triad', suggesting that these are emergent states that arise from the interaction between three main neural systems. These are the emotion-valuation; sensory-motor; and meaning-knowledge systems (Chatterjee & Vartanian 2014). Neuroaesthetics is a fast-growing field of cognitive neuroscience that aims to study the neural foundations and mechanisms of aesthetic experience, predominantly through non-invasive brain stimulation (Cattaneo 2020; Pelowski et al. 2017; Nadal & Skov 2015; Chatterjee & Vartanian 2014). Aesthetic experiences are known to engage the default mode network (DMN) in the brain (Belfi et al. 2019; Vessel et al. 2019), which is generally activated when individuals are involved in self-referential processing (Cattaneo 2020). The functions of the DMN also include 'daydreaming' or 'mind wandering', which is similar to the sense of 'flow' that the sensory nature of clay and art work in general encourages. Creating one's body image from clay, which engages self-referential processing and flow, would therefore activate the DMN, a reward centre of the brain, enabling feel-good hormones to be released (Lesage & Stein 2016, p.25).

In their fMRI analysis of aesthetic responses to art, Vessel et al. (2012, p.1) identified two diverse patterns of neural activity from different brain sub-networks, firstly, a sensory occipito-temporal region associated with visual processing, and secondly an area of the frontal regions belonging to the DMN – involved in self-referential thinking. Vessel et al. (2012) suggest therefore that aesthetic experience involves 'the *integration* of sensory and emotional reactions in a manner linked with their *personal relevance*' [our emphasis]. It has also been found that *self-referential* material enhances the recall of memories (Kelley et al. 2002, p.785). Therefore, by co-designing body image sculptures, full of personal relevance, it is likely that the intensity of the aesthetic experience felt by the women involved in the study was increased (Vessel et al. 2012), enabling the development of a positive mood and the attachment of *emotional resonance* towards the sculptures, and by default, themselves.

How we judge a work of art is to some degree dependent upon how much personal resonance it engenders, as indicated when we view images or sculptures of people, with which we have a shared embodiment and human-ness. As Gallese (2017, p.7) claims '[. . .] other types of MMs (mirror mechanisms) underpin our capacity to directly apprehend the emotions and sensations of others because of a shared representational bodily format'. This means that our human-ness means we are able to 'experience others as experiencing emotions or sensations we know from the inside [. . .]' (ibid.).

Research carried out by Shohamy & Wagner (2008) demonstrated that making connections between disparate events activated the hippocampus, associated with memory, and the neurohormonal midbrain regions, associated with the release of dopamine a (feel-good) chemical that acts as a neurotransmitter, particularly associated with identifying and moving towards a reward. This indicates that making new associations and linking diverse phenomena may trigger the reward centres of the brain. This suggests that an increase in positive affect may be achieved by increasing *broad* rather than *narrow* associative processing in healthy individuals (Bruyneel et al. 2013). Therefore, therapeutic interventions that broaden clients' capacity for associative processing may be beneficial for clinical disorders such as post-traumatic stress disorder (PTSD), anxiety and depression, and obsessive-compulsive disorder (OCD) (Bar 2009).

Embodiment, Empathy, and Clay Work

Perceiving and handling objects that exist in the world, such as clay sculptures, engages our visual and sensory perception, which utilises a 'bottom-up' neurological process driven by *sensory stimulus* from the outside world. This interacts with a 'top-down' internal *cognitive* process, driven by expectation and goals (McMains & Kastner 2011, p.587; Hass-Cohen 2008, pp.31–32). The main task of the visual system is to provide the brain's higher cortex with a coherent representation of the environment, so that *sense* can be made of it, and this sense-making is mediated by emotion. Both top-down modulation and bottom-up stimuli have been found to activate the amygdala (emotional mediators in the brain), although bottom-up *sensory* processes have been found to elicit a *stronger* response (Ochsner et al. 2009, p.1322), suggesting the emotive power of sensory visual art such as body image sculpture.

When judging the 'beauty' of nude bodies, the anterior cingulate cortex and the nucleus accumbens areas of the brain are activated (Martin-Loeches et al. 2014), and these are the same areas of the brain that are active when assessing the aesthetic value of figurative sculptures and objects of art (Di Dio et al. 2011; Calvo-Merino et al. 2010; Cattaneo et al. 2015 & 2017; Cazzato et al. 2014 & 2016; Ferrari et al. 2018).

The discovery of 'mirror neurons' is also important when considering empathy and body image, as Rizzolatti et al. (1996) highlight a direct link between empathy and imagery, revolutionising the way automatic physical responses to sensory images (seen directly in life or in art) are understood. This has contributed to the knowledge that human beings possess a 'body-based understanding of the world' (Gallese & Lakoff 2005, p.466). Gallese et al. (2002, 2005) called automatic physical responses to sensory images *embodied simulation*, which translates to a person's capacity for automatic responses that *imitate* others' physical or emotional states, suggesting that discursive knowledge, or verbalization, is not required for the 'empathic matching of experience' (Gallese 2006; Hass-Cohen 2008, p.304). Therefore, the same neural networks are activated in the brain when viewing a person in pain (in life or in a sculpture), 'as if' the viewer was also in pain (Keysers et al. 2004), meaning that we not only *recognise* the pain of others, we also *embody* others' emotional states (Carr 2014, 2018).

Embodied simulation also works when metaphors are verbalised; therefore, when a metaphor involving an action verb is used, e.g. 'to grasp a concept', the regions in the brain involved in motor perception and physical action around the word 'grasp' are activated (Samino 2010, p.202). Similarly, a metaphor such as *a velvety voice* activates the areas of the brain associated with the sensory tactile experience of velvet (ibid.).

The neuroscience behind *imagination* has also shown that when imagining or visualizing something, the activity shown in the human brain resembles that associated with the real experience (Buckner & Carroll 2006), suggesting that 'imagined phenomenon are not just a *figment of our imagination*, they are part of our *embodied experience*' (Carr 2014, p.65). Clay work offers an embodied way of working through body image issues, with movement, gesture and sensory qualities offering a *bottom-up* neurological process for psychological change. This bottom-up embodied process, is highlighted by the human development of using our hands for fine motor skills, something which has been fundamental to the shaping of the modern human brain (Wilson 1998).

Within this chapter we have discussed recent neuroscientific and neuropsychological research as an explanatory tool for the effectiveness, and sensory processes of clay work within art therapy, as well as neuroscientific studies which begin to explain why an altered perception of body image occurs in eating disorders (ED). Recent neuroscientific studies that have highlighted the effect of emotion on vision, aesthetics on emotion, and the link between embodiment and metaphor, were also discussed. The premise of this chapter was that by exploring published neuroscience research which underpins sensory and metaphorical processes employed in clay work, knowledge and understanding of the subject will be increased. This will also be used to underpin findings in the case studies and the concluding chapter.

Section 2

Vignettes and Case Studies – *Shaping the Self*

4 Case Vignettes, Study One

Sessions One, Two, Three, and Four

Study One, Session One: Helena, Sarah, Victoria, Linda, Veronica, and Nancy

Within this chapter, case vignettes drawn from Study One of Dr Trisha Crocker's PhD research project exploring the use of clay work as a tool for exploring body image, are presented. Sections from a *reflexive diary* written by Dr Crocker for the duration of the study are also referred to. Images of the clay body image sculptures created by the women involved in the research project, and transcripts of voice recordings of the women talking about their experience of creating the sculptures, are used to highlight and discuss the themes found in the analysis.

Helena

Helena was 42 years old at the time of the study and identified as British/Asian. She was married, and at the time of the sessions, her daughter was soon to be a teenager. Helena was brought up in the UK by her English grandmother, her parents were divorced and living in Asia. Helena had a post-graduate degree in fine art, and spoke openly to the group about having experienced two late miscarriages.

Helena engaged herself completely in the clay work process and shared freely within the group. After the clay work the group took part in a general discussion about the clay body image sculptures they had made and the process of building them. At the beginning of the discussion, the participants seemed a little reticent about speaking within the group; however, Helena again initiated the dialogue by discussing body size and attitudes around the world. She talked about how in Victorian times women were expected to wear suffocating corsets and some even had operations to remove their lower ribs, in order to gain an hourglass figure.

For Helena, the process of creating her body image (see Figure 4) involved using the clay to make body modifications, including 'covering over':

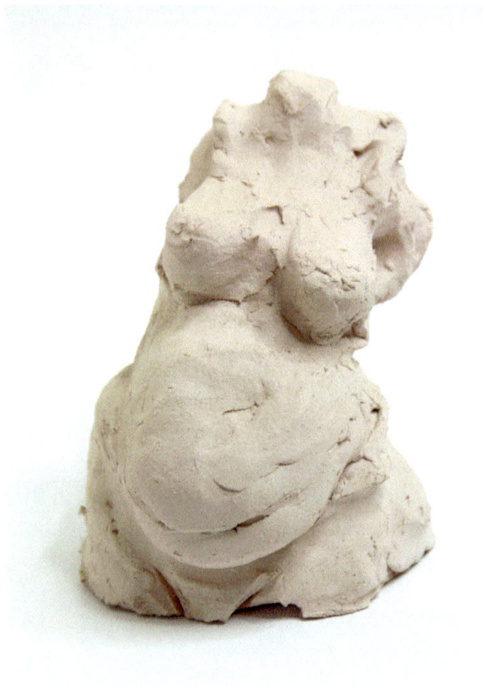

Figure 4 Sculpture No. 1 by *Helena*.

"I'm Ready Just to Cover That Over."

> "And it was really amazing to be able to cover it over with clay, literally you know, the physical process of being able to, sort of, see some shapes that you want to keep and some shapes that you think 'no', I'm ready just to cover that over. I think that's incredibly satisfying, which I didn't expect."
>
> *Helena*

Art Therapist/Researchewr Reflective Diary

I reflected that perhaps Helena uses the word 'cover' to explain how she 'covered over' parts of herself that she disliked, meaning that she no longer needed to think about them. Because of Helena's wholehearted engagement with the clay work and the discussion, it seemed that Helena was willing to consider her feelings on a deeper level, and gain personal understanding through the discussion and clay work.

Helena described the group session as "compelling, emotional, and gratifying" and described how the time spent making her body image enabled her to realise that reflecting on her body image through clay work – although at times painful – could help her come to terms with the losses she associated with her body image.

Sarah

Sarah was a 48-year-old woman who identified as white British. Sarah was divorced, and a mother of two primary school age children, and also working as a Doctor. As Sarah was a single working mother at the time of the study, she talked about how she was forced to juggle her life around her children and her work. Sarah engaged without hesitation in the making of her clay sculpture (see Figure 5), and instead of focusing on her body image in a realistic way, she chose to reflect on her body and inner self through metaphor and symbolism.

> "Yes, I've got no body. I'm running though, which is me all the time. I've got my arms wrapped around my – well, my three heads. Me, my mummy head, and my work head."
>
> *Sarah*

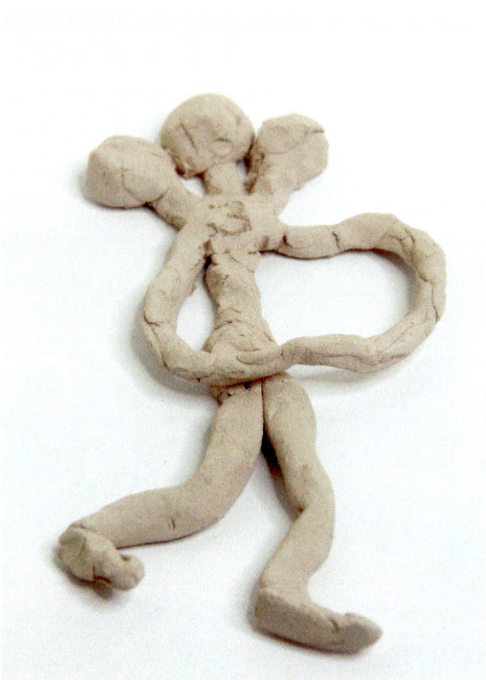

Figure 5 Sculpture No. 1 by *Sarah.*

"Me, My Mummy Head, and My Work Head."

Art Therapist/Researcher Reflective Diary

I reflected that Sarah's sculpture utilised metaphor and symbolism and seemed to show her being 'pulled in all directions', having to 'be' many different identities at once, meaning that she lost sight of herself as a whole person, becoming instead a collection of disparate, but individually functioning 'parts'.

Sarah's second sculpture was similarly focused on aspects of her body image rather than the 'whole'; using metaphor and symbolism again, she referred to this sculpture as a "Smile on a Stick". (see Figure 6)

Art Therapist/Researcher Reflective Diary

After representing herself as a 'smile on a stick' Sarah spoke to the group about how she felt about her body. I had noticed that Sarah was distressed while making the 'smile on a stick' clay sculpture, finishing about 20 minutes before the others and going off by herself to make a cup of tea.

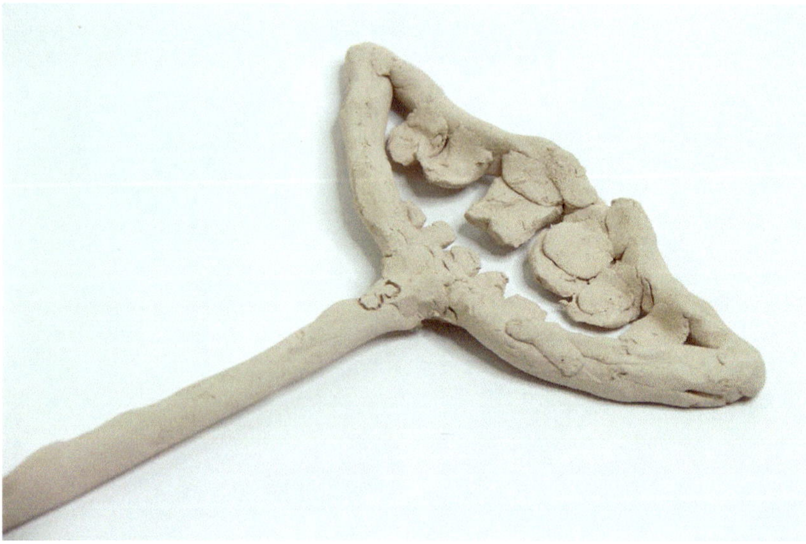

Figure 6 Sculpture No. 2 by *Sarah*.

"Smile on a Stick."

Sarah explained to the group that there was pain behind the 'smile' as she was often criticised because of her naturally tall, thin body. Sarah spoke of an incident at the gym when she had the uninvited appraisal of an older man, who told her bluntly that her body was 'unattractive'.

In the group discussion, it seemed that Sarah wanted to speak about what her sculptures represented but was tearful and seemed conflicted about divulging more within the group situation.

Art Therapist/Researcher Reflective Diary

Within the group I acknowledged to Sarah that the discussion appeared to be difficult for her. Acknowledging Sarah's discomfort allowed the group time to reflect on the difficulty of speaking out and to understand that no one would be urged to speak if they were not ready. I also wanted to make sure Sarah left the session feeling supported, and with her concerns acknowledged.

Victoria

At the time of the study Victoria was 48 years old, a white British woman, who was divorced and a mother to two adult sons. Victoria had recently been trained and employed within a county borough as a family/child worker.

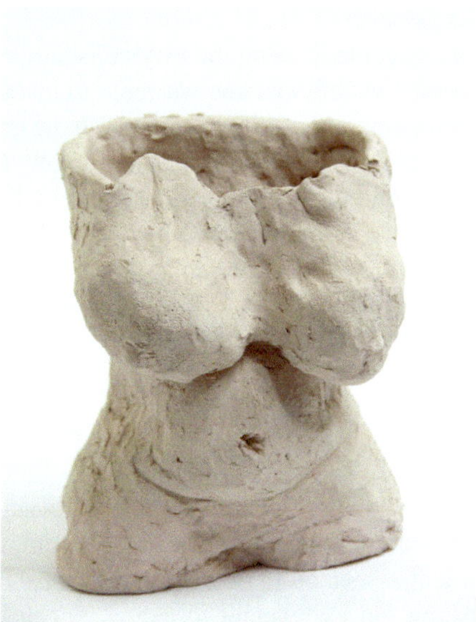

Figure 7 Sculpture No. 1 by *Victoria.*

"Victoria's Concern About Her Large Breasts."

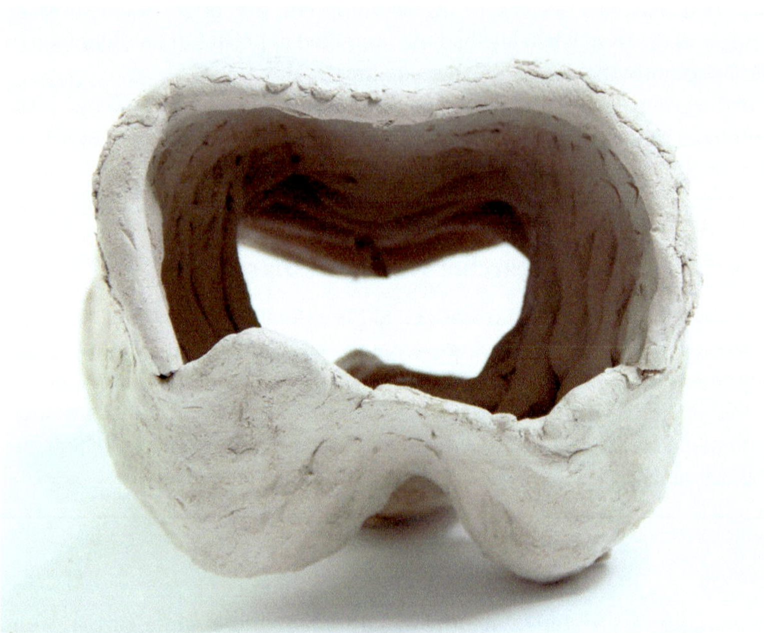

Figure 8 Sculpture No. 1 (from above) by *Victoria.*

"A Large Hollow"

Victoria made her body image using the clay coil-building method and then smoothed the coils out, meaning that she was able to make her sculpture hollow. When it was Victoria's opportunity to share with the group, she was asked by one participant if there was a reason it was left hollow and she replied that this was how she had been taught to make a sculpture when in school. Leaving a large hollow in the form made it *container-like* when looking into it and seemed to emphasise the size of the breasts. Victoria expressed concerns about her large breasts and said she wanted to have her 'athletic and healthy body again', but she told the group that her 'weight' affected this desire.

Art Therapist/Researcher Reflective Diary

I reflected on whether the 'hollow' or 'container-like' nature of Victoria's sculpture might represent something else, such as emptiness or incompleteness. Victoria also seemed to be suggesting that she was in a 'catch 22' situation, feeling too overweight to exercise. The 'emptiness' may therefore represent feelings of loss – regarding her 'athletic, healthy body' that she feels she has lost – and also guilt, at feeling unable to change this.

Linda

Initially Linda seemed to struggle with making her body image from clay; however, in the end she produced three, very different sculptures. Linda also used words such as 'wall', 'cover', and 'protective cover' to describe her first image (see Figure 9). Although Linda struggled to find herself in the image, these three words spoke volumes about Linda's effort to 'cover' and protect her embodied self behind a 'wall'.

> "This here, that I started to do, actually – believe it or not, it's the spine. I've got quite a few issues with the spine here. And it's funny I should do this first, because I made it almost like – you know – like a sort of wall, really. The idea was I was going to put my body into it, but it didn't really go. And it's almost as . . . I've used it as . . . a wall. As, like a cover, which . . . comes across . . . why I probably couldn't get into it, because the first thing I started to do was, like, this protective cover around me, and I think that's what I've done. So, I really couldn't get into myself. It's strange . . ."
>
> *Linda*

Linda told the group during the discussion that her daughter often told her she was 'too heavy' but that she herself wasn't necessarily 'worried' about being heavy unless it affected her health.

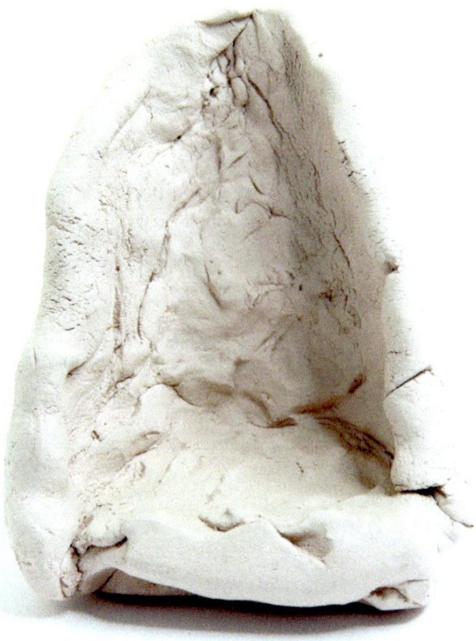

Figure 9 Sculpture No. 1 by *Linda.*

"It's the Spine."

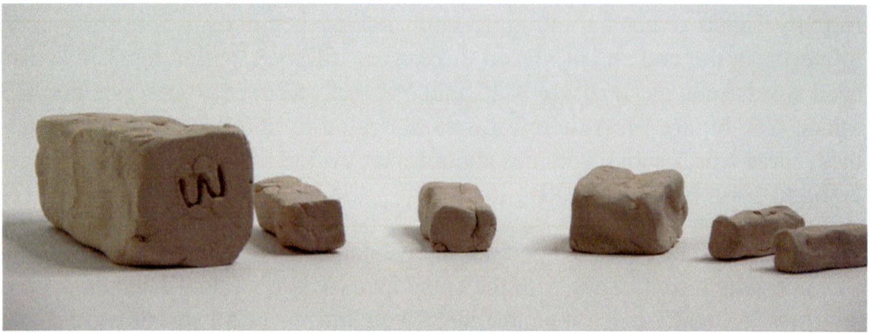

Figure 10 Sculpture No. 2 by *Linda.*

"All Women."

Linda's second image was abstract and symbolic; however, she explained that it was a metaphor for 'all' women (see Figure 10). The image was made up of rectangular clay blocks of differing sizes that, when laid out in a certain way, Linda said were representative of a body. Again, Linda struggled to find herself in the image, which may have demonstrated that for Linda, focusing on her body image, except as an abstract form, was difficult.

Art Therapist/Researcher Reflective Diary

I wondered if Linda's sculpture "All Women" represented all women as objectified 'parts', or all women as 'in pieces', divided up into abstract objects such as the head, breasts, legs, bottom etc. Because the session allowed for only a certain amount of discussion time for each participant it was not possible to take this further within the group. I was aware that it was an opportunity missed. This was one of the frustrations of being in my 'researcher' identity and sitting in on the group as an observer rather than as a therapist.

Linda's third and final sculpture, entitled "Gosh, I don't even think I've got a body . . ." (see Figure 11), demonstrates that Linda was perhaps beginning to recognise how she had dissociated from her body in the past. However, as she worked through this, she began to create a 'figure-like' sculpture and get in touch with her body through the clay work saying that she was aware of feeling 'quite choked' when she worked on her third sculpture.

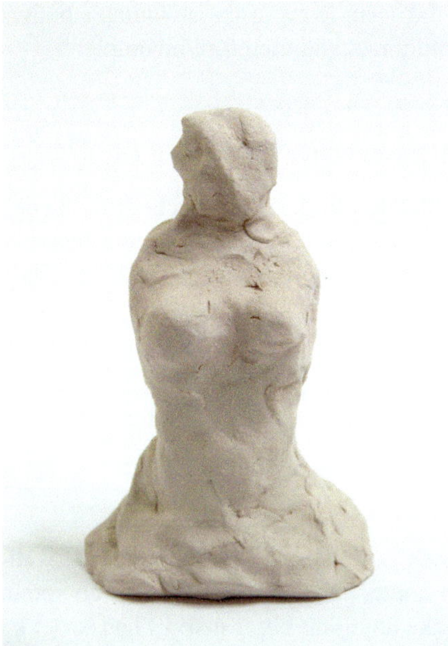

Figure 11 Sculpture No. 3 by *Linda.*

"Gosh, I Don't Even Think I've Got a Body!"

> "Gosh, I don't even think I've got a body, which was quite a bizarre thought really. Quite disturbing, really."
>
> *Linda*

Art Therapist/Researcher Reflective Diary

I wondered if the feeling of being 'choked' indicated a psychological obstruction that blocked Linda from reflecting on her body within the first two sculptures. As a therapist, I would have liked to pursue this further with Linda; however, the time constrains of the study, and the necessity of ensuring that all the women left the session safely, meant that this was not possible. On reflection I believe that the one-hour discussion provided enough time for contemplation, without allowing room for anxiety to build that could not be addressed. Rather, the women were given the opportunity to reflect and recognise that they all shared similar doubts and insecurities about their body image. (The women were all made aware that further one-to-one art therapy including body image clay work was available outside of the study had the women wished to pursue this.)

Even though Linda declared "I don't even think I've got a body', this third and final sculpture did seem to represent a woman's body, although it was just the head, breasts, and torso, and therefore incomplete.

Art Therapist/Researcher Reflective Diary

I reflected that although important aspects of the body were missing in Linda's third sculpture, time may have been a factor in this. It seemed that Linda was making progress working with the clay and beginning to get in touch with her body.

Veronica

Veronica spoke about deliberately making a wall before she could create her body image.

> "Yeah, I couldn't do anything until I'd made a wall. It just wouldn't – nothing would come, and I was wanting to do something big, but then, I don't ever make anything big. I just – I had to – I kept playing with the clay, thinking you know, I've got to – something's got to appear out of this. And then once I'd made this, sort of, protective space, I thought, oh, now I know what I'm going to do. And it just – the idea came."
>
> *Veronica*

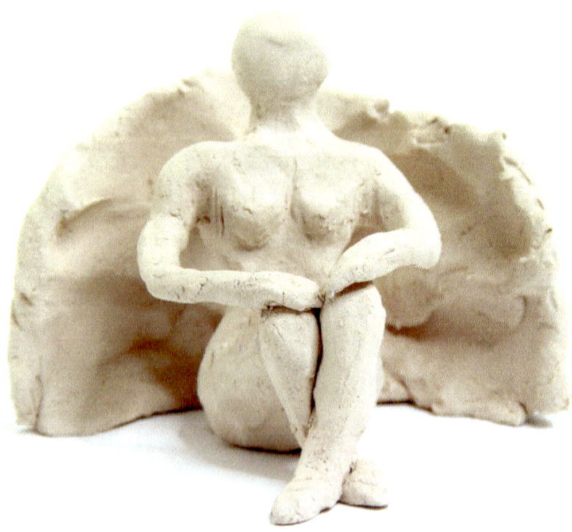

Figure 12 Sculpture No. 1 by *Veronica*.

"I Couldn't Do Anything Until I'd Made a Wall."

One participant suggested, "It is very closed down here", pointing to the lower half of Veronica's body image sculpture (see Figure 12), "very guarded". Veronica replied: "We've all had some spinal connection, be it that it's a protective thing or that it's a flexibility thing, or that it's more root."

During the group discussion Veronica was asked what she had been thinking when she was making her body image and what feelings were brought up for her as she worked.

> "I felt really exposed doing it. I couldn't make . . . I couldn't . . . I thought, I'm not doing anything out of this clay, and then, once I'd made a protective space, I could make something inside that."

Linda explained that the 'wall' in her body image sculpture had not initially been built as a wall, but as part of a 'spine', and Veronica's 'wall' emerged behind the image. However, both 'walls' seemed to offer a form of protection for the women, something they needed to create before creating their body image.

Art Therapist/Researcher Reflective Diary

I wonder if there was a subconscious connection found by the women between the safe therapeutic space and the protective space mentioned above that allowed for further exploration. Also, a 'wall' can indicate a boundary, barricade, fortification, impediment, hurdle, or façade, suggesting that some interesting double meanings may also be going on here. Again, these double meanings would have been explored further had there been time.

Nancy

At the time of the study Nancy was a single 34-year-old white British woman, working for a UK borough council as a trained child/family worker. Nancy engaged enthusiastically with the clay work, whilst trying to be 'honest' about her body image issues (see Figure 13 on p.62).

> "Yeah. For me, it was about being really honest. I, kind of – I think since probably the beginning of this year, I've been on a bit of a journey with my body. So, there's part of me that looks in the mirror every morning and says, Yeah, it's alright. It's not too bad. It's okay. It's liveable. I can go out and do stuff. And the other part of me is really self-conscious about it, and I think – I mean – I've been going through, probably, through the last couple of months being very honest about things and opening up, sort of, matching what was going on in my head to what I was actually saying, and

> sharing with people about how I am uncomfortable, and all of those kinds of things. So, for me, today, it was about [saying] 'No, this is my body.' I have to be honest about it. There's part of it I don't like – I have an image of what I would like to look like and how I would like to be. But I am not sure that my body matches up with who I think I am in my head, if that makes any sense."
>
> *Nancy*

"In my head" appeared often in the discussions and reflections and was usually begun or followed up with an exclamation stating "it sounds silly" or "it might not make sense to the listener". This may indicate an awareness that describing their 'body' from 'in my head' is a contradiction, or at least demonstrates a tension between a cognitive 'brain based' understanding of the body or an embodied 'felt' understanding.

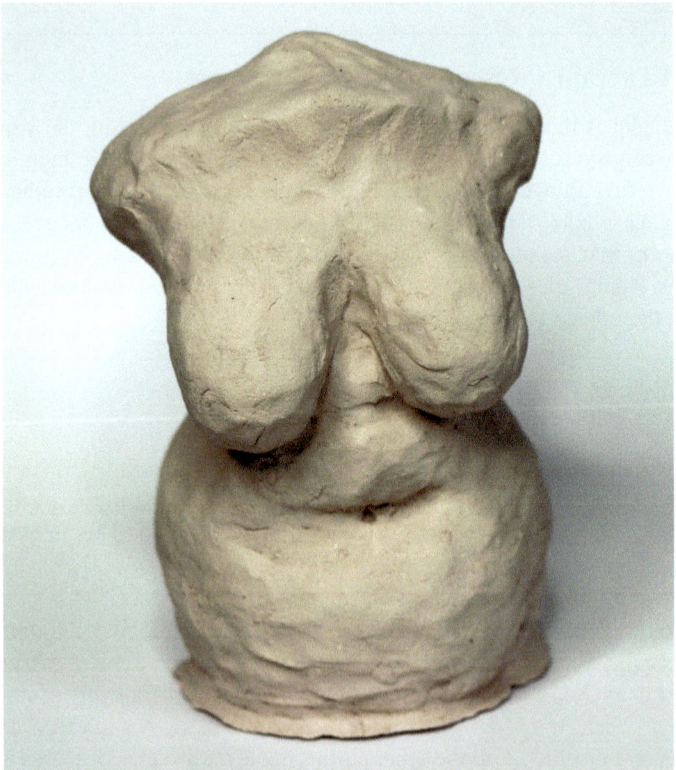

Figure 13 Sculpture No. 1 by *Nancy.*

"For Me, It Was About Being Really Honest."

Art Therapist/Researcher Reflective Diary

After the session I reflected that Nancy was one of those who contributed the most to the discussion. She also appeared one of the most relaxed in the group and with the clay work, and therefore seemed willing to consider her feelings on a deeper level, and obtain personal understanding through the manipulation of the clay.

Study One, Session Two: Jenny, Edina, Willow, Priscilla, and Jane

Jenny

At the time of the study Jenny was 44 years old, a white British woman, married and a mother to two adopted primary school aged children with special needs. Jenny had previously held a high-powered job when she had met her husband. Together they owned a large house in the country. Jenny was also a carer for her parents, who were unwell and lived a long distance away.

Jenny's body image sculpture was a female torso on a round plinth, with additional detached rounded segments (see Figure 14).

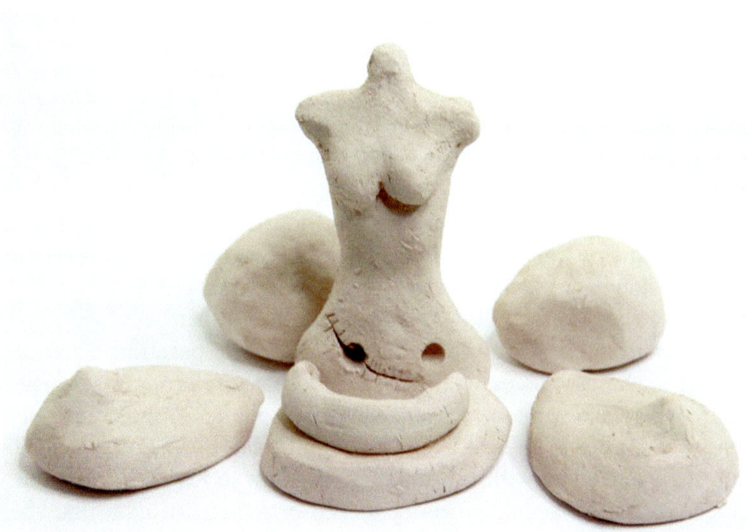

Figure 14 Sculpture No. 1 by *Jenny*.

"I've Got a Comfort Layer. . . ."

Jenny had inscribed 'scars' on the torso, front and back. The front scars, she told the group, related to her kidneys. Jenny spoke about her body having 'segments', which were the pieces of her body image sculpture that were left unattached to the torso:

> "And because of that I've got a comfort layer, which I've grown, which is these enormous boobs and these buttocks actually, my bum, and rolls [of fat] which actually, if I'd been showing you, that sort of has to fit on there. Because it all covers it up quite nicely. And that's what I've morphed into, but because I've done it . . . that . . . people don't ever see my face anymore, as far as I'm concerned. It's really interesting, because you've got a lovely shape and you can think about your face, whereas I tend to think people don't see my face. I'm invisible now. I'm just a blob."
>
> *Jenny*

Feeling 'invisible' is a common issue highlighted by women as they age, with women feeling that they are no longer seen or validated by society for who they are (Hurd & Griffin 2008). Feeling invisible can impact on a person's body image and body-esteem. For Jenny, body image and body-esteem are two different things:

> "I say that body image for me is something that's a very practical thing and something that can be very manufactured. Body-esteem involves the mind."
>
> *Jenny*

Jenny spoke at length about her mother's views on being a woman in her own generation and her need to always look and be the perfect wife for her husband. One of the participants said that her mother was from an era where a woman felt she had to look and be perfect for her husband, always wearing lipstick, being smart and tidy, and a showpiece for the man. This prompted a long discussion on past and present views on body image.

Jenny then revealed to the group that she 'hated' her body and how this stopped her from enjoying trips with her husband to beautiful places in the world where he associates with beautiful people, preferring instead to stay at home where she wouldn't be judged. Jenny said her husband had told her seven years earlier that she was unattractive because of her size, something which she said stayed with her and added weight to her belief that she was unattractive. She spoke of their courtship and explained that at the time she had been very slim. Jenny spoke of her sadness around having miscarried a baby and being unable to conceive again, which prompted them to adopt two small children with special needs.

Edina

At the time of the study Edina was 41 years old, and identified as a white British woman, and mother to two sons. Edina was working as a florist and was married to an artist.

Edina told the group that she was born into a family of 'larger women', which made her 'hate' her own body, saying she had struggled with her weight and a negative body image for many years, and felt defensive about her size. Edina said she had lost two stone and kept it off for quite a long time, but was still worried about how she felt about herself when she was with her family.

Edina's body image sculpture had emerged as a figure that was immobile, on its knees, and therefore unable to move (see Figure 15). Without legs, and with arms joined together across her breasts, there also seemed to be a general lack of 'agency' in the sculpture. The sculpture also had no facial features, so was in addition 'deaf,' 'blind', and 'mute.'

Art Therapist/Researcher Reflective Diary

I reflected that Edina's sculpture with missing body parts may have been an unconscious indication of her struggles around maintaining a positive body image.

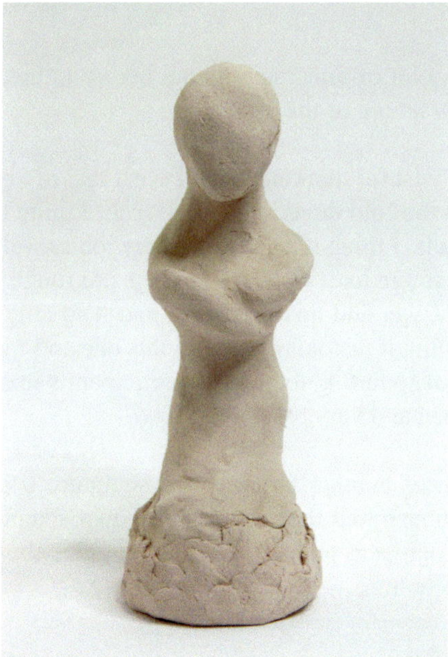

Figure 15 Sculpture No. 1 by *Edina.*

"I Think I Feel Quite Defensive About My Size at the Moment."

Edina spoke about why she had recently chosen to take action and lose weight:

> "I must admit I did struggle with how I'm feeling mentally, and as people see me, and the struggle to differentiate between that. I think it's because I'm so crabby at the moment. Hence the defensive pose, I think. I think I feel quite defensive about my size at the moment. Coming from a family of larger women I always feel I have to justify my size. It's taken me a while to get [down] to this size because I don't want to look like them, which has spurred me on, absolutely. I did struggle with that really, yeah, definitely."
>
> *Edina*

Art Therapist/Researcher Reflective Diary

This led to a lively discussion on how to lose weight within the group. I eventually had to curtail this and bring everyone back to a safer place, as the remarks - although meant as helpful - appeared to be aimed specifically at Jenny, who I felt was quite vulnerable after speaking about her sculpture and body image issues.

Edina had spent a lot of time 'smoothing' her sculpture, indicating that she enjoyed the sensory nature of the clay.

> "I think that's wishful thinking. That I wish that my body was somewhat smoother than the 'old duvet' that it is. Yeah, I quite like smooth. I don't know why that is. I think it's because of my job as well, where everything that I touch is rough and, well, most things are rough and slightly mucky and, you know, wet and this is smooth and it's really nice. Yeah, I don't know why. I think it just felt right with this one and I wish I could convey myself like *that* [pointing to another participant's image], because it just seems very open and very relaxed." *Edina.*

Edina's admiration of another participant's sculpture being 'very open and very relaxed', demonstrated that she felt her own sculpture was lacking in these qualities, recognising perhaps that the struggles she went through were played out in her sculpture.

Willow

Willow was the youngest participant in the group sessions at only 25 years old, and a slim, fit, personal trainer. Willow had not yet experienced motherhood

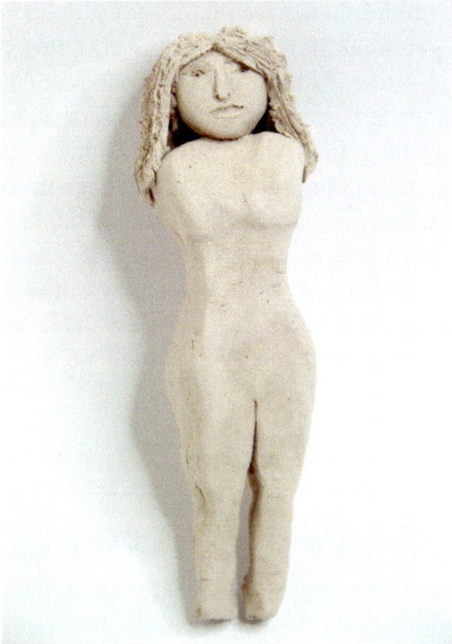

Figure 16 Sculpture No. 1 by *Willow.*
"The Face Was Most Important."

and the body changes that pregnancy can bring. However, Willow had spoken about how her mother had undergone many operations to change the shape of her body in different ways.

Art Therapist/Researcher Reflective Diary

I noted that the subject of 'manufactured body image' e.g. cosmetic surgery, was not taken further by the group during the discussion. Although there had been a lengthy discussion between all the participants regarding their own interpretations of body image and body-esteem.

Willow spent the first half of the one-hour clay work session concentrating on sculpting her head and hair, and creating a detailed face (see Figure 16). She later made a flat, rather featureless body to stick the head onto, but kept returning to the head and face in order to refine it. Willow's body image was also incomplete, in that limbs and connecting body parts were missing, e.g. neck, arms, hands and feet. The body also appeared androgynous, with no distinguishing female features.

> "I think for my part – I don't know if it's the same for you, but the reason I had lots of definition in the face is . . . I just don't . . . I think probably because when you think how people view you, that's the first thing they see and that I also like. I didn't put any arms on or I didn't really worry too much about the legs, because I don't think when you look at someone, that's what you look at first. You tend to just look at, you know, the shape and the outline, and so I probably shouldn't have thought what other people are thinking, but you can't help it I don't think, when you do something like this. But I naturally wanted to portray myself, sort of, as I think people would look at me for the first time, as well as what I, in the mirror, worry about and look at. You know, those are the things I look at, not, you know, is my arm long enough or, you know?"
>
> *Willow*

Art Therapist/Researcher Reflective Diary

I reflected on how Willow was a 'sporty' personal trainer and yet claimed that she 'didn't think of her body', but about 'her face' and how others see her. Perhaps Willow felt that as a personal trainer her face was less easy to alter than her body, or perhaps she had no issues with her body? The featureless, androgynous shape of Willow's body image sculpture also reminded me of a 'mannequin dummy,' used in shop displays.

It seemed that being young (only 25 years of age) and lacking in body-changing experiences such as childbirth and parenthood might have been a factor in Willow's lack of engagement with her body image. There may also have been an unconscious belief that if her body image was a problem, she could follow in her mother's footsteps and have surgery to 'correct' any issues. In attempting to create a 'perfect face', or a good model . . . Willow may have been seeking acceptance from the other 'older' women in the group. These issues would have been areas to pursue had there been time.

Art Therapist/Researcher Reflective Diary

On reflection I acknowledged that although many younger women do experience body image issues, it was important to purposefully select older women for Study Two, in order to focus the project more and draw boundaries around the study.

Priscilla

At the time of the study Priscilla was 51 years old. Priscilla identified as a white British woman, was married and a mother to three teenage girls. Priscilla said the family did not own a television for the majority of her children's school years so that their childhood would not be exposed to outside influences that she and her husband would be unable to control, saying that as parents, they wished to give the children a wide variety of skills and interests both inside and outside of the home. Priscilla had worked as an engineer before having her children.

Priscilla had made it clear from the beginning that she was attending the session in order to work on her body image, and had already been thinking about this before she arrived. Priscilla invested a great deal in the session, which gave her the space to explore the many body image issues she brought to the session.

Priscilla was determined to begin creating her sculpture as soon as she arrived, and did not appear interested in the courtesy of introductions, which made the atmosphere in the studio somewhat tense initially. The powerful imagery that Pricilla created in the session was also a lot for the other participants to take in, particularly for those who were more tentative in their approach (see Figure 17 and Figures 18 & 19 on p.70).

Using a sharp clay tool to inscribe angry, frustrated words into her body image ensured that they were not hidden or difficult to read, suggesting that Priscilla was determined to express her pain and face her body image issues within the group.

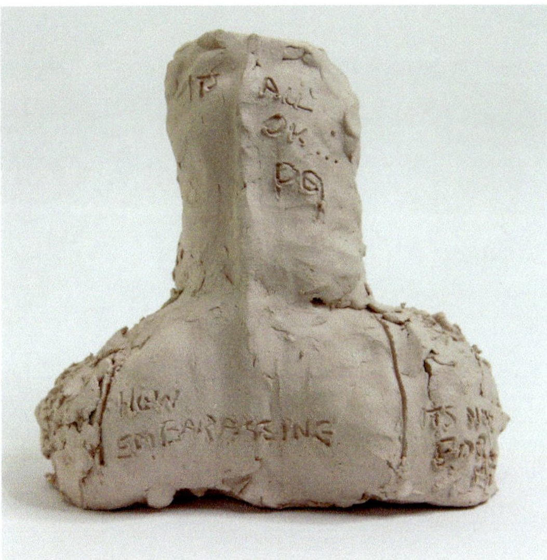

Figure 17 Sculpture No. 1 (Front) by *Priscilla*.

"How Embarrassing."

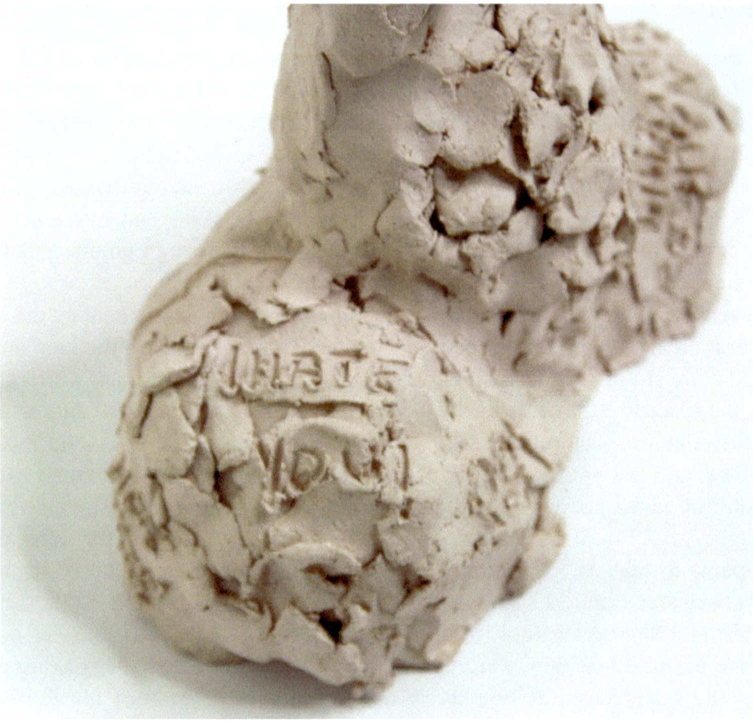

Figure 18 Sculpture No. 1 (R. Side) by *Priscilla.*

"I Hate You."

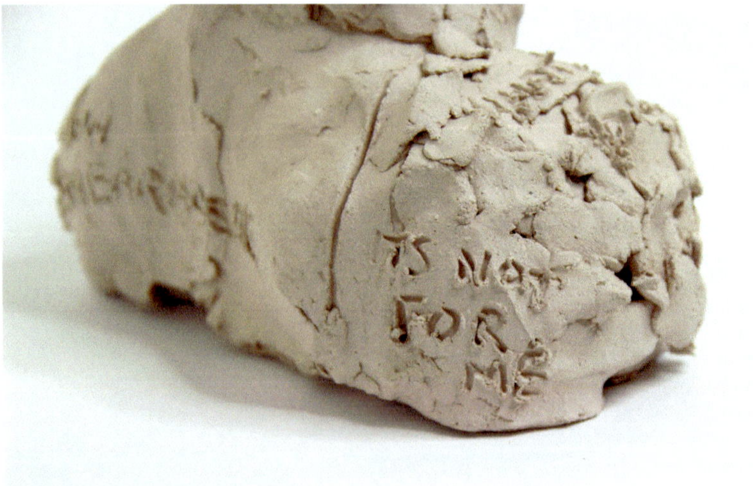

Figure 19 Sculpture No. 1 (L. Side) by *Priscilla.*

"It's Not for Me."

Art Therapist/Researcher Reflective Diary

I wondered if Priscilla had expected all the participants to have an equivalent loathing of their own bodies. This helped in the decision to make Study Two individual rather than group sessions, and to invite Pricilla to be part of it, so that she could explore further the long term and major issues she had with her body image.

Priscilla's sculpture was very powerful and demonstrated a lot of courage in exploring this among the other participants. However, the fact that the other women were also exploring their body image, and were (mostly) strangers, may have made it easier for Priscilla to openly confront her issues. Priscilla's sculptures are discussed further in Chapters 5 and 6.

Jane

At the time of the study Jane was 57 years old, married, a mother to one teenage son, and also a teacher of profoundly handicapped children. Jane was one of only a few participants who created a full body image sculpture, which she said was about reminiscing memories of her younger self, and "remembering what it felt like to do the splits" (see Figure 20). Initially Jane was frustrated about her lack of clay work skills:

> "This sort of frustrates my lack of technical skill, which I know is completely irrelevant, but it still frustrated me – that I couldn't actually do what I wanted to do."
>
> *Jane*

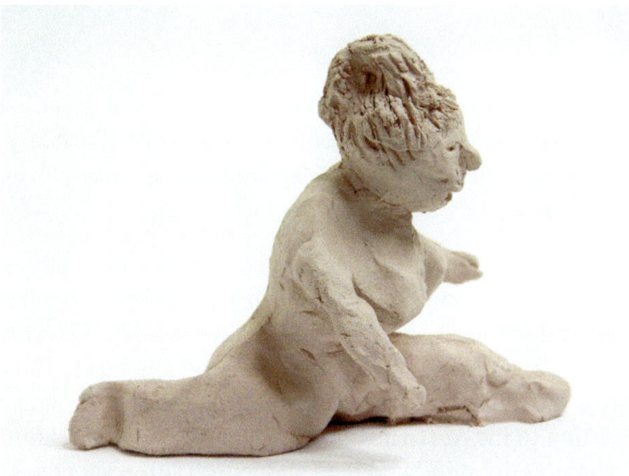

Figure 20 Sculpture No. 1 by *Jane.*

"Remembering What It Felt Like to Do the Splits."

Jane continues by talking about being "close to retirement" and aware of her aging body:

> "But . . . I suppose I was, coming to a transition of . . ., so coming close to retirement, aware of an elderly body, beginning to suffer from mechanical failure and a real need. But I can't actually, you know . . . I can't actually move like that though, so, I mean there's a need for that . . ."
>
> *Jane*

Written Communication from Participant: Jane

> *Jane said that the discussion was "thought provoking" and that she was surprised by the discussions that developed and how open everybody was. Jane said she felt very stimulated by the session and that it highlighted the group's "humanity".*

Art Therapist/Researcher Reflective Diary

I reflected that the session was at times painful, and at times angry, but there remained a sense of humour within the group as the women grasped the fact that they had so much in common. They also showed a lot of empathy for each other and spent a lot of time trying to build each other's confidence through supporting their feelings and seeing a positive in the images. This is perhaps a positive factor for brief group work in art therapy/research; the support of each other through the common bond of womanhood can be of great benefit. However, whilst individual work can be more intense, it has the benefit of safely delving deeper into the recesses of memory over an extended period of time.

Eleanor

At the time of the study Eleanor, was 47 years old and identified as white-Canadian, she was married, and mother to a boy and girl of primary school age. Eleanor engaged well with the clay but became emotional as she explained her sculpture (see Figure 21):

> "My image has three distinct but connected parts. My body is flanked by my head (my mind), and by my heart (my emotions). The three appear to be 'equal' but the head and the heart chain the body. The chain entwines the body and is a direct link between my head and heart. The emphasis in the body is intended to be the arms – reaching, stretching, and growing out of proportion to the rest. The phrase 'trying to throw her arms around the world' came to my mind and then suddenly I felt tears come to my eyes. The head has a serene and happy face but there are traces of tears on it. The heart is whole, solid, unbroken . . . a story."
>
> *Eleanor*

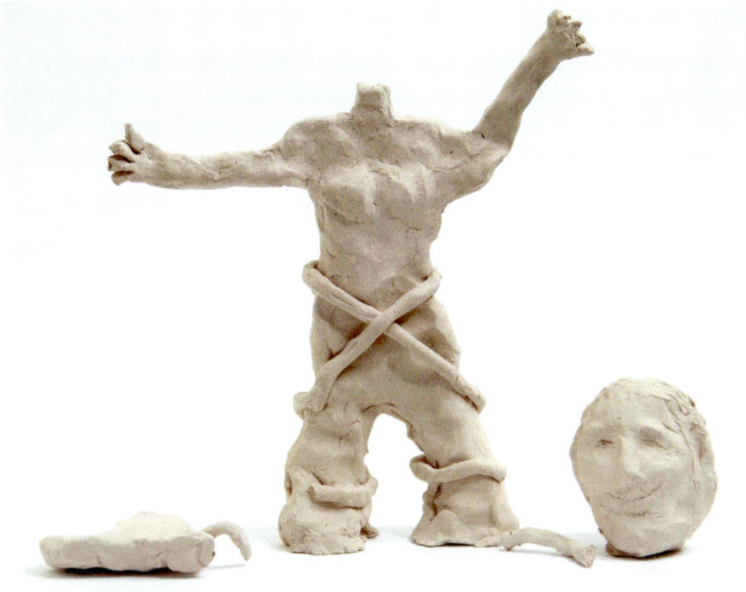

Figure 21 Sculpture No. 1 by *Eleanor.*

"Three Distinct but Connected Parts", or "Broken Pieces."

Eleanor's sculpture was similar to Sarah's sculpture "Me, My Mummy Head, and My Work Head" (see Figure 5 on p.53). For both women there appeared to be a need to embrace the family as well as their jobs; perhaps this was what was happening when Eleanor mentioned and felt emotional when saying the words "trying to throw her arms around the world".

Missing body parts and an inability to 'see the body as a whole' is another theme which began to emerge in the images of Sarah, Linda, Jenny and Eleanor. There was also a sense of 'fragility' in how they were constructed.

Art Therapist/Researcher Reflective Diary

After the session, when I carefully moved Eleanor's pieces still on the board to the drying area, the 'chain' broke. This affected me deeply and I wondered how such a flimsy chain could have been expected to remain intact. It suggested to me that perhaps there was more to Eleanor's story than discussed on the day . . . and there was. Eleanor wrote to me from Canada a while after the session (see below).

Post-Session Written Communication from Participant: Eleanor

> "Curiously, I don't identify myself as a mother, although of course I have two children and I love and admire and like them very much. I see myself as a supporter of their growth to independence; a fosterer of their development as people; and I hope I am a role model for how to live well."

Art Therapist/Researcher Reflective Diary

I felt that many questions were left unanswered by this statement, yet perhaps it is just Eleanor's straightforward thoughts on herself as the mother of her two children. It left me wondering what her own mother's role was in Eleanor's childhood, until she wrote again to me ostensibly on the subject of body image, though so much more came to light.

Post-Session Written Communication from Participant: Eleanor

> *"My parents were not parent-like: they were not role models, they did not act in our interest, they were primarily absorbed in their own drama, they did not encourage us or take much notice of us [. . .]. So . . . body image? It is important to me to be natural and to be comfortable with myself [. . .]. Maybe because my mother and sister were so concerned with their attractiveness to men and because that was clearly their territory, I simply took another direction. . . . "*

The separation of the head from its body in Eleanor's sculpture, correlates with the other 'headless' sculptures produced by participants, and perhaps indicates feelings of disembodiment, or dissociation from her body. Eleanor states that the 'head' has a 'serene and happy face'; however, she qualifies this by stating that there are 'traces of tears on it', acknowledging that there is pain within, despite her heart being 'whole, solid, unbroken . . . a story'.

Paula

At the time of the study Paula was 39 years old, a white British single woman with no children, working as a primary school teacher and hypnotherapist. Paula spoke of struggling with the 'weight' of the clay and having some technical difficulties around building her sculpture (see Figures 22 & 23). Paula also said that she had not knowingly used metaphor or symbolism in its construction.

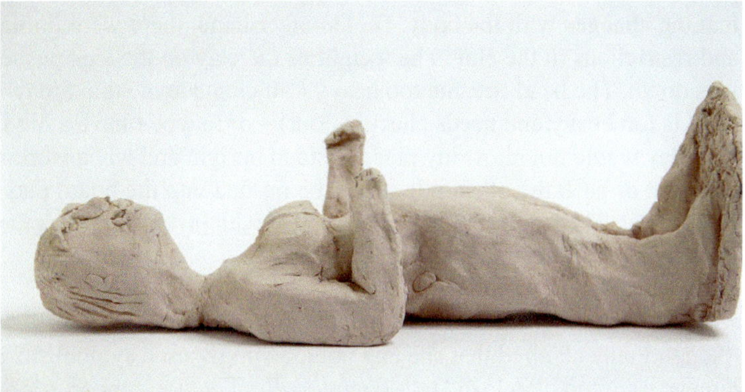

Figure 22 Sculpture No. 1 (Front) by *Paula.*

"The Image Is As I See the Outside World Seeing Me."

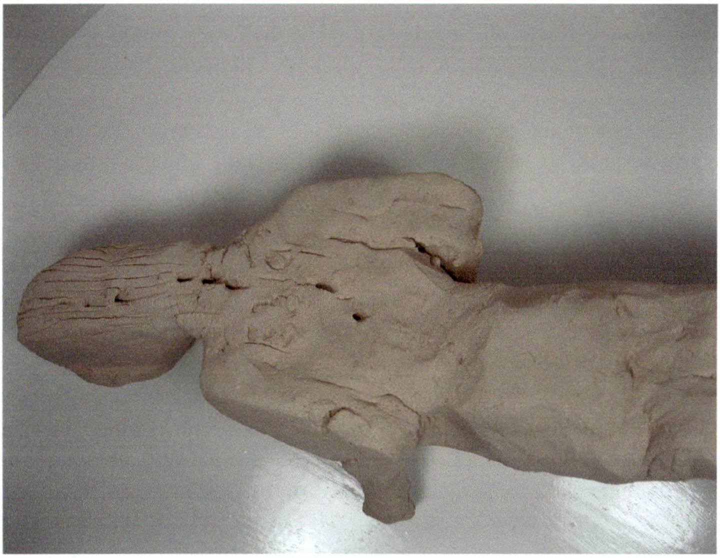

Figure 23 Sculpture No. 1 (Back) by *Paula.*

"Like a Piercing."

"The image is as I see the outside world seeing me. There is no imagery or symbolic element. Although there are aspects which do not quite fit with how I see myself due to the restrictions with the clay use, the weight of the body pushed down onto my legs making them shorter, fatter, and stumpy. I considered if this is how I saw my legs in my head but realised it was not so pronounced and became a little frustrated with the weight pressing down onto the legs – I could find no solution. The clay had a soothing texture and feel, which made managing the image pliable – a little like making changes with the body. On the other hand, there were limitations and restrictions to the clay. The weight of the clay on the legs pushed the legs down. The head became too heavy (which made me think maybe my head is too heavy and needs checking out) – or maybe I have a big head? The clay would not allow my piece to stand upright and when working on the front or back the other side would be pushed into the board making it more squat. The support of the model ended with [a] stick coming through the clay to the other side – like a piercing!"

Paula

Although Paula claimed that she had not knowingly used symbolism in her body image sculpture, Paula did talk *symbolically* about the support stick coming through the 'skin' of the torso, saying it was like a 'piercing'.

Art Therapist/Researcher Reflective Diary

I wondered if Paula was ready to explore her body image at this time of her life, or prepared to reflect sufficiently to make changes. Perhaps she felt unable to explore any deeper due to the restraints involved in a one-off session and/or the presence of others. This reminded me of the requirement to be sensitive to clients' needs, and remember that not all women are ready or able to reflect on their body image within a group.

Justine

At the time of the study Justine was 47 years old, married, mother to two boys of primary school age, and also working as an editor.

Justine used a combination of realism and symbolism within her body image sculpture which revealed important information about her own dreams and personality, as well as herself and her family (see Figures 24 & 25). Justine described the metaphor and symbolism within her sculpture in great detail:

"The image represents me – absorbing and caring. The smooth piece in the circle is me – the calm part that allows me to absorb and also to consider my response and reflect. The curved wings around the hollow are me enfolding things in care. The pearl in the smooth part of the hollow is my husband and the recognition that I am very fortunate to have this strong presence and love in my life. The overall shape is how I think of myself – very feminine. The spine represents a strong backbone, both independent and able to carry others. The little people are the fun I have with family and friends and my sons. The book represents my dreams and aspirations. The hair represents my vanity – it is important to me to look the best I can and my hair is important to this. The hair also represents wings."

Justine

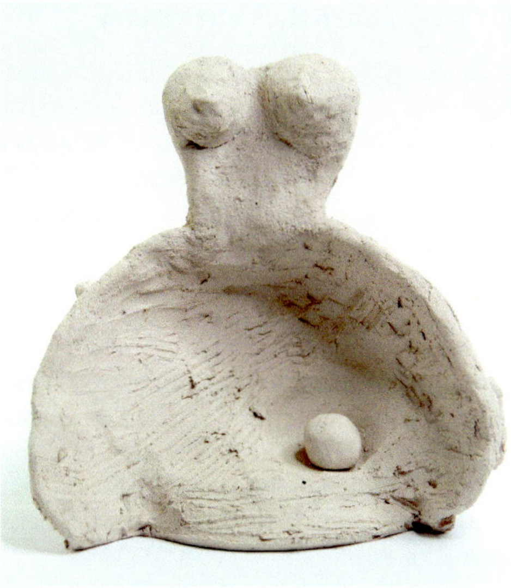

Figure 24 Sculpture No. 1 (Front) by *Justine.*

"The Pearl Is My Husband."

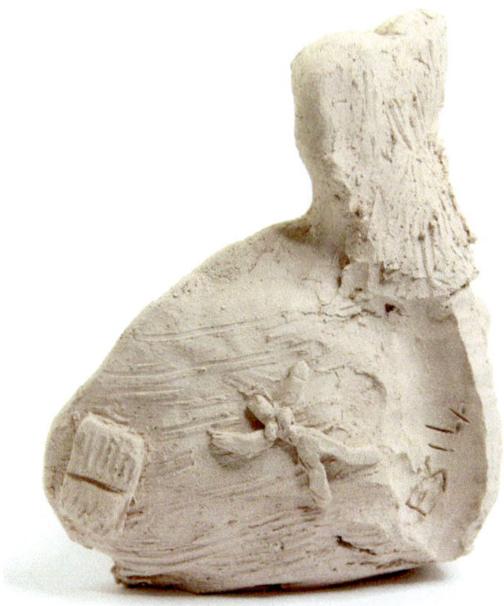

Figure 25 Sculpture No. 1 (Side) by *Justine.*

"The Spine Represents a Strong Backbone."

Art Therapist/Researcher Reflective Diary

I reflected that Justine gave a very personal interpretation to the words; smooth, wings, hollow and backbone. Several of these words were used by other participants when describing their body image sculptures; however, all were specific to their particular image.

Sunny

At the time of the study Sunny was 41 years old, and mother to three primary school aged children. Sunny identified as British/Asian, was born in India, was married to an English man, and had worked as an engineer before she left to become a full-time mother. Sunny listened intently to the other women in the group. Sunny's interpretation of her body image (see Figure 26) was similar to Justine's, who had also focused on her role as a mother when creating her sculpture (see Figure 25).

Sunny said that although she heard the instruction to 'create your body image in clay', she proceeded to make what appeared to be a boat, with herself and her three children inside of it.

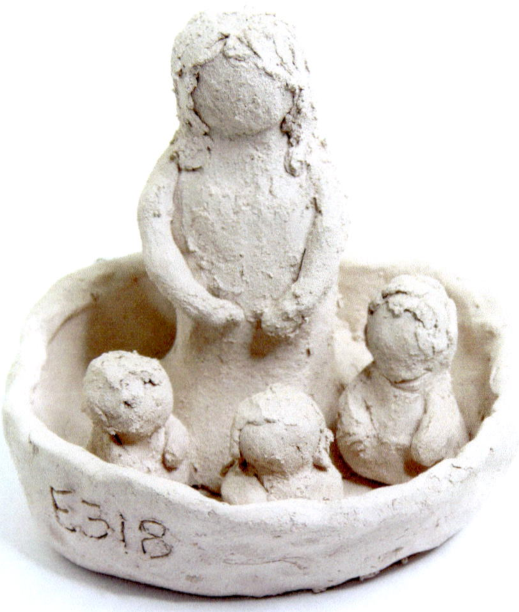

Figure 26 Sculpture No. 1 by *Sunny.*

"I Think the Image Represents Me as a Mother."

"I think the image represents me as a mother since that is my most defining role at the moment. I guess I would like the image to convey a woman who has had three children. I hope it represents my feelings of contentment and completion, which is probably how I feel about my family. . . . Actually, I feel that I do not have very strong feelings about my body image other than wishing to be healthy. My body image is far more defined by the fact that I have been pregnant. My body shape has changed since having children. I no longer feel the need to think a great deal about my outward appearance."

Sunny

Art Therapist/Researcher Reflective Diary

I wondered if this might reflect a cultural divide . . . where the female body may be thought of as something that primarily exists to attract a husband and produce children although this may also be prevalent in Western culture too.

Sunny was very much a part of the group discussions, although she had little to say about herself and her body image except that she was a mother and just wanted a healthy body. It seemed that Sunny was unable to separate her body image from that of motherhood.

Cynthia

At the time of the study Cynthia was 52 years old, and identified as a white British woman. Cynthia was a trained nurse and a mother to two adult children. She had been separated from her husband for a number of years, but due to necessity they were still living in the same house.

In this sculpture by Cynthia (see Figures 27 & 28 on p.80) she seemed to present herself as a 'wizened owl,' 'stuck' in over-large trousers. Cynthia explains in her own words what the sculpture and the clay work sessions meant to her:

Written Communication from Participant: Cynthia

"My head is perhaps the 'inside' of me; my body the 'outside' and creating a body image was, therefore, for me about my external body rather than my internal one. It's my slim and sensual side trying to take flight from all the 'baggage' and weight I carry with me. My wings are my hands too . . . reaching out – my creativity – looking for someone to pull me out/rescue me. I am stuck. My face – my jowls – I hate the fact my face is growing saggy! But as I made the skin/jowls they became part of an owl's face. My wisdom has replaced my youth! – sort of. My breasts and neck and upper torso I like. My arms are trapped but my hands are trying to reach out from the back."

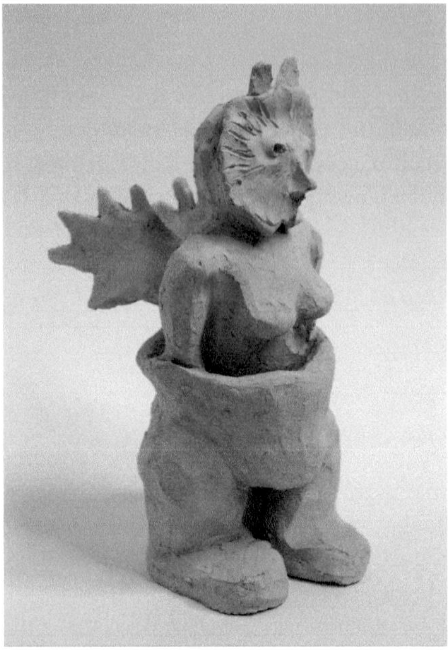

Figure 27 Sculpture No. 1 (Front) by *Cynthia.*

"As I Made the Skin/Jowls They Became Part of an Owl's Face."

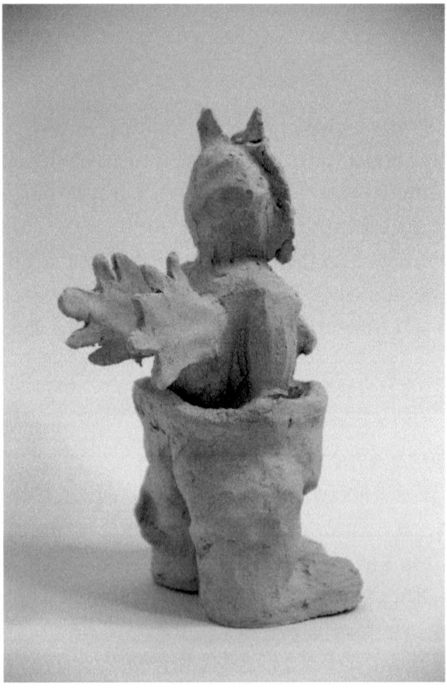

Figure 28 Sculpture No. 1 (Side) by *Cynthia.*

"My Wings Are My Hands Too, Reaching Out."

Post-Session Written Communication from Participant: Cynthia

> *"Thank you for the leg up! There is a reason for my constant search and questioning and now I seem to be reaching some kind of summit! Funny . . . after my session with you I felt v. vulnerable in a 'new' way, not a negative way, and as my therapist so rigorously spotted 'well . . . you've lost your trousers! Indeed, I think I left them in your studio!"*

Cynthia talks of the pay-off of aging, where she says that her *youth* has been replaced by *wisdom* and further recognises the usefulness of the clay work she has done, saying she is "well on the way out of those trousers". The 'trousers' may be a metaphor for Cynthia's perceived lack of femininity.

Post-Session Written Communication from Participant: Cynthia

> *"I feel very honoured to have been a subject and also very curious! I still think the work I did with you was very helpful and am well on my way out of those trousers and finding some that fit better and also reveal my femininity!"*

Within this session metaphor and symbolism were used intuitively by the participants, adding meaning and significance to their clay sculptures. Metaphor and symbolism are generally an important part of art therapy work, and something that clay work has enabled within this study.

Study One, Session Four – Sunny, Justine, and Cynthia

Sunny, Justine, and Cynthia were invited to attend another clay body image session, as they appeared to be very comfortable and relaxed in each other's company despite none of them knowing each other prior to the group. This fourth session was set up to further refine the questions and other considerations needed for Study Two, and to enable the women to explore their body image further.

Sunny

In Session Three, Sunny made what appeared to be a 'boat', 'container' or 'enclosed wall', holding herself and her three children (see Figure 26 on p.78), telling the group that she had focused on herself as a mother, rather than on her body image *per se*. This previous session perhaps provided a sense of safety and gave Sunny 'permission' to be more forthcoming about her body image in this subsequent session. Sunny also became engrossed in listening to the stories of other participants and engaged more fully in the discussion.

> "I was probably influenced a little from the last session. I really wanted an upright image of myself. I would hope the image represents myself as satisfied and in control of myself (hopefully not in a smug way). I am not bodily perfect but I hope the image conveys I still feel feminine and basically that I still like my body despite the changes that have occurred due to age. I think the positive about the image is [it's] quite a proud one."
>
> *Sunny.*

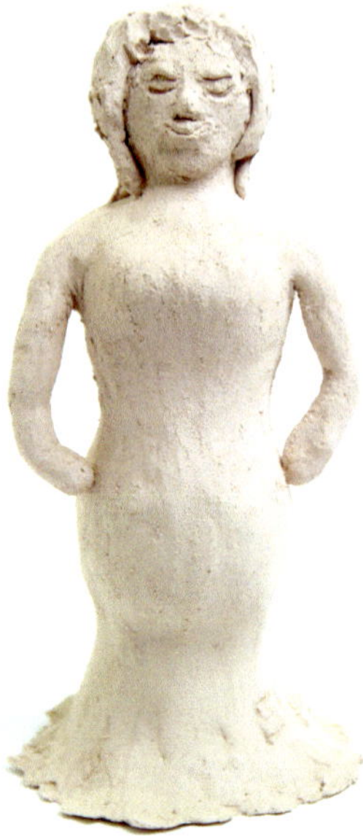

Figure 29 Sculpture No. 2 by *Sunny.*

"I Think the Positive About the Image Is It's Quite a Proud One."

Art Therapist/Researcher Reflective Diary

I reflected that Sunny felt comfortable within the session as she now knew and liked, and perhaps trusted, the other members of the group. Sunny may therefore have felt equipped emotionally to make an attempt at creating her body image from a different perspective.

Sunny told the group that she was happy with her upper body and therefore this was where she began the sculpture (see Figure 29). Sunny said she wanted her body image to be 'symmetrical and with a very straight back and with smooth lines.' Sunny also said her hair was important to portray as well as her 'rather large features'. Sunny appeared to enjoy the shared discussion and responses and support that the other group members offered.

Sunny's body image sculpture (see Figure 29) was one of only two body images created during the study where the figure is wearing clothing, in this case a dress, the other being Cynthia's 'trousers'. This 'covering' of the body with a 'dress' was not spoken about by Sunny, nor did the group members question it.

Art Therapist/Researcher Reflective Diary

I wondered if perhaps Sunny's Asian background influenced her decision to keep her body covered. Perhaps Sunny would have felt shame or embarrassment with regards to revealing her naked body. However, I noted that Sunny appeared to feel comfortable and at ease in both sessions as the women spoke of their bodies and the personal issues raised by them.

Justine

Justine attended the fourth session having spent time thinking about how she would like her body image sculpture to represent her and talks about her second sculpture (see Figure 30 & Figure 31 on p.84):

> "It was important for me to try and make the body proportions as 'lifelike' as I could – if any part was too large or too thin as I perceived it, I wasn't happy and reworked it until I felt it was a fair representation. I thickened the waist to represent my thickening middle and made my bosoms slightly droopier, with one lower than the other as this is how they are. It was important for me to try to work the 'behind' accurately – I spent a lot of time trying to get my buttocks right and my legs in some way shapely. The odd lumps and bumps represent my some-way shapely aging body."
>
> *Justine*

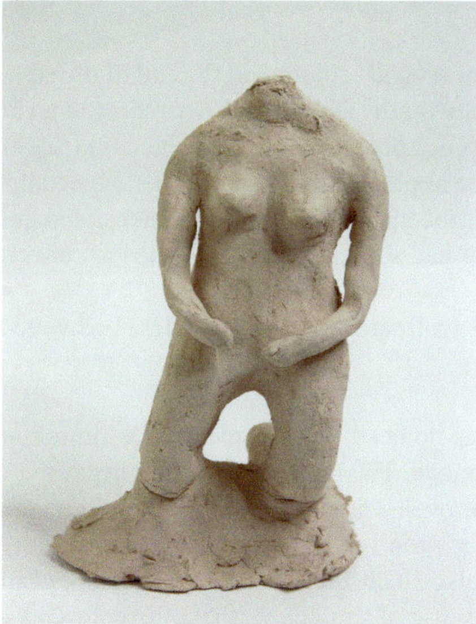

Figure 30 Sculpture No. 2 (Front) by *Justine.*

"The Odd Lumps and Bumps Represent My Some-way Shapely Aging Body."

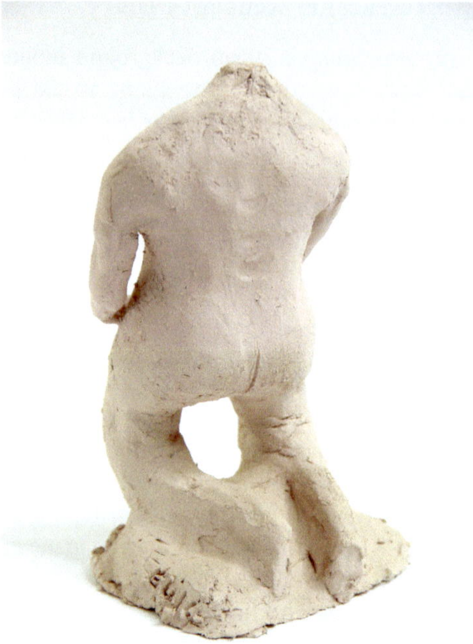

Figure 31 Sculpture No. 2 (Back) by *Justine.*

"I Spent a Lot of Time Trying to Get My Buttocks Right and My Legs in Some Way Shapely."

Writing about her second sculpture at the end of the session, Justine said she was able to connect with the clay to help her reflect in an honest way about the changes she saw in her body. Justine said she could see the changes that age had brought, yet she appeared able to adjust her expectations. Justine said that the tactile nature of the clay, with its three-dimensional quality, was important as it meant that she had something of substance to reflect on, rather than just a memory.

Justine's second sculpture was also 'headless', as were several of the other women's sculptures:

> "The image has no head – it was clearly less important to me than creating the body image. The image is kneeling because I needed to anchor it, so it didn't fall over – doing this made it look like it was up to her knees and stuck. This wasn't at all what I wanted to portray, so I modelled her kneeling – I also liked the freedom of movement this gave the image. I also like the sense of suppleness that this represents – it is an acceptance of the body – an ease with the body which I like. I still think her bottom is too big . . ."
>
> *Justine*

Art Therapist/Researcher Reflective Diary

What came across when listening to Justine was her honesty about the changes that were taking place in her body due to age, and her efforts to accept these as a natural part of growing older and maintain a positive outlook.

Cynthia

In this session Cynthia made a round shape and hollowed it out and then placed another round ball with a hole on top inside the hollow (see Figure 32). Cynthia used a sponge and water to smooth the surfaces of her shapes. As she talked about her image with the group, they all showed intent interest, but appeared to be taken aback initially by Cynthia's honesty and the resemblance of her sculpture to female genitalia. However, they seemed to identify with much of what was said, expressing concern that – within a Western culture – much of what women feel about aging and the intimate parts of their bodies, is often left unsaid.

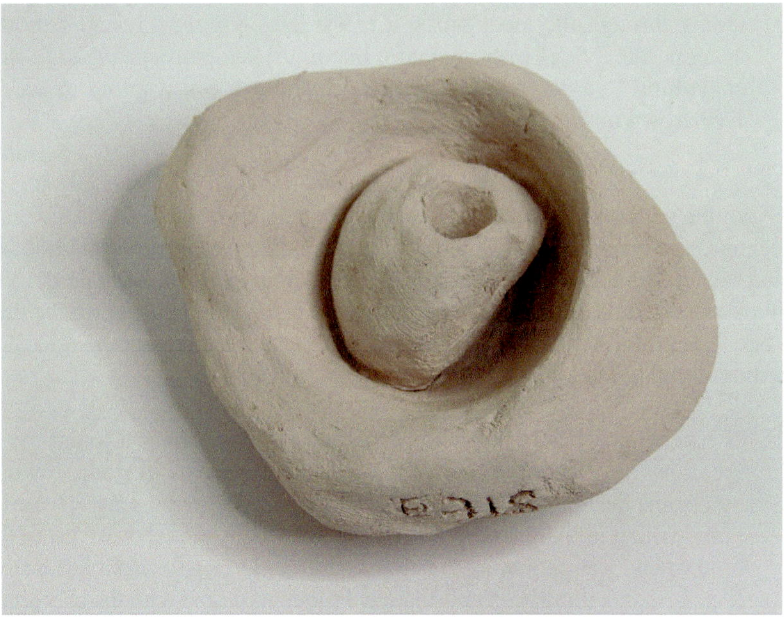

Figure 32 Sculpture No. 2 by *Cynthia.*

"I Felt Sadness and Almost Tearful when I was Scraping Out a Hollow Within Myself . . . My Womb?" or "The Mushroom Shape."

Art Therapist/Researcher Reflective Diary

I wondered if being of the same gender and similar ages gave the women in the group 'permission' to be more candid when talking about what it meant to be a more mature woman, and the women in the group intuitively explored the image and its resemblance to female genitalia, with Cynthia.

Cynthia explains the process of creating her sculpture:

> "I began with a large clump of clay, I wanted a solid piece focusing on my present feelings about my body. I felt quite nauseous at one stage and this changed significantly when I worked on a small inner part of my sculpture, like I was attending to it and soothing it. I felt sadness and almost tearful when I was scraping out a hollow within myself, my womb? My children? Abortions? Loss, not of use, my age, lack of sexual loving relationship, mourning old past relationships. Using my body, abusing, letting it be abused, I felt protective of what is left. The overflowing muffin hangover on my middle seems like a protective layer. Going through the menopause, a crossroads, ending – fear. I hate the spare part that flops over my jeans, like in the sculpture, trying to fit into something I've outgrown, wanting to fit into it. Not wanting to accept I've grown up."
>
> *Cynthia*

Cynthia's account of her image was one of reflection and a flow of words, feelings, and questions. Cynthia mentioned childhood trauma but did not discuss this in detail. Although she had not practised in the art therapy field, Cynthia understood the art therapy process and became very engaged in the clay work. The sculpture seemed to open a door to Cynthia's private thoughts and feelings, whilst also allowing others in to discuss them.

> "I became attached to the mixture of good and bad parts and found pleasure in learning that my negative bits are in fact positive in some way and hold some meaning. The clay felt comfortable, yet I felt a sense of 'struggling' with it initially, and some frustration. I really enjoyed the rest of the time when I was beginning to make the form – I yearn for what lies inside. It enables transformation and change. I thought of food with the clay slip – the chocolate cake mixture my mother used to make."
>
> *Cynthia*

Part of Cynthia's written response at the end of the session again validates the importance of *trust* in a group therapy session:

Written Communication from Participant: Cynthia

> *"We seemed to gel in the other session, which was lucky. I was very pleased to be asked to be in the same group again. It would have been something to consider if asked to continue. It would have been interesting to see how my work would have been with new people. I felt more trusting and quite comfortable with being open."*

Cynthia enjoyed playing with the clay, saying that the wet slip mixture reminded her of chocolate cake mixture. The clay work gave Cynthia the opportunity to explore her body image, and access past memories that opened up new channels of exploration and unlock a lot that she held within. The clay work also enabled Cynthia to explore her body image from inside to outside, opening a path to engage further with her past. Because of Cynthia's enthusiasm and willingness to uncover, explore and understand her past, as well as her ability to be open to discussion, Cynthia was invited to participate in Study Two.

Art Therapist/Researcher Reflective Diary

I reflected that although working with the wet slip clay reminded Cynthia of a chocolate cake mixture, other participants remarked that it reminded them of faeces – and therefore may have been an indication of regression and getting in touch with their child/baby selves. Had this been an on-going group, this might have been a useful topic to explore with the group in more depth.

Themes Identified Within Study One

The eight main themes identified from Study One sessions were:

No.	*Theme*	*Potential Meanings*
1.	'Covering', and 'building walls' and/or 'containers'	Shame, hiding and protecting the self and body image.
2.	'Dissociation' from the body	Feeling a lack of 'ownership' of the body or lack of 'embodiment,' or not feeling 'at home' in their own body.
3.	'Missing' body parts	Not feeling 'whole' as a woman, the body being a sum of 'parts'.
4.	'The critical mother', and 'motherhood'	Attachment and embodiment issues.
5.	'Aging', the changing body and feeling 'invisible'	Lack of control over body changes, and over 'being seen' or 'not seen'.
6.	'Anger, loss and sadness'	Mourning losses.

(*Continued*)

(Continued)

No.	*Theme*	*Potential Meanings*
7.	'Shared humanity, experience and compassion'	Recognising that other women in the group shared many of the issues raised by individuals. Feelings of solidarity and empathy regarding this.
8.	'Sensory nature of clay' and 'smoothing'	The properties of clay offer a sensory, calming, soothing, experience.

In Sarah's first image, "Me, My Mummy Head, and My Work Head" (see Figure 5 on p.53) and Eleanor's "Three Distinct but Connected Parts", or "Broken Pieces" (see Figure 21 on p.73), both women chose not to focus on creating a realistic body image sculpture, but instead concentrated on how they felt about themselves symbolically and the roles their bodies fulfilled (e.g. being a mother, working etc.). This may reflect the way in which they heard the instructions, or it may be that they felt the main significance of their bodies was as a mother and worker. This demonstrates the versatility of clay work, enabling the use of metaphor and symbolism and/or realism, both in the actions used to create the sculpture, and in the form it takes.

Both Eleanor and Sarah enjoyed positive feelings of self-esteem from their work and had young children who demanded a part of them that they were eager – but stretched – to give. Creating body image sculptures that did not feature a recognisable 'body image' may also suggest feelings of 'dissociation' from their bodies, perhaps linked to feeling a lack of 'ownership' and a need to 'find yourself again'. Veronica, one of two women in the session who also identified as a 'stay at home mother' (and was in a process of change regarding her primary relationship), reflected on Sarah's sculpture "Me, My Mummy Head, and my Work Head" (see Figure 5 on p.53):

> "When you're a 'mum,' I think you forget there is a 'you.' You are just a mum. If you've got a job, then you've got a job. If you're just a mum, you're just a mum, until – well for me, until they started moving into their teens, you then start to find 'yourself' again."
>
> *Veronica*

Art Therapist/Researcher Reflective Diary

I reflected that Veronica suggests women may not focus on their own body image as a major issue when they are wrapped up in family and work, in that ". . . you forget there is a you". However, it is important to remember that a lack of time to focus on their own body image does not mean that these women have no body image issues, and that these issues may resurface once their children leave home, or if their relationship breaks down, etc.

The clay-making allowed for these thoughts on motherhood, work, and body image to surface and gave the participants space to think about who they were, how they perceive themselves, and how they were perceived by others.

The theme of sadness and loss regarding body image was brought to the fore for some of the women through the clay work. Jane spoke about losses relating to her body in "Remembering what it felt like to do the splits" (see Figure 20 on p.71), saying she had once been athletic and fit, and embodying this fitness within her sculpture. Jenny also identified losses to her body image when discussing her sculpture "Broken Pieces" (see Figure 21 on p.73), saying she had once been slim and fit through running and going to the gym with her husband when they were first together.

The theme of covering the body, or building a wall to 'hide' behind, suggests feelings of 'shame' or anxiety around body image. Veronica's sculpture embodied these feelings as she first built a wall for her body image sculpture to 'hide' behind, saying "I couldn't do anything until I'd made a wall [. . .]", calling it a 'protective space' that she needed to build before she could create her body image sculpture. Linda struggled to make her body image from clay, but when discussing the three sculptures she created Linda used the words 'wall', 'cover', and 'protective cover' to describe her pieces and the process of making them.

In Justine's image "The Pearl is my Husband" (see Figure 24 on p.77), Justine's 'wings' with a 'strong backbone' also became the sheltering, protective 'wall' seen in Veronica and Linda's body image sculptures (see Figure 12 on p.60 & Figure 9 on p.57). The word 'backbone' was also used to explain strength in Linda's "It's the Spine" sculpture (Figure 9 on p.57) where the 'vertebrae of a spine' was built into the 'wall'. The group also referred to Victoria's sculpture (see Figure 7 on p.55) as having a "strong backbone". The need to 'cover', or 'build protective walls' around one's body image speaks of an acknowledgement of 'vulnerability' as well as a sense of 'shame'.

The nature of the clay, and for some the struggle to construct their sculptures, also brought various issues to the fore. Justine used the word 'stuck' to describe difficulties she experienced while constructing her sculpture (see Figures 30 & 31 on p.83 & p.84), in particular, determination to make her figure stand up. Paula also had issues regarding this, but instead allowed her body image sculpture to recline (see Figures 22 & 23 on p.75). The word 'smooth' was also used by the participants throughout the sessions and discussions, often referring to the sensory nature of handling clay, and wanting their body image sculptures to be 'smooth' even though they knew their own bodies were 'lumpy' and 'bumpy'.

Using group clay work sessions for study one meant that the women involved were able to create and discuss their body image on an equal plane, and offer support and compassion to the other women, and also receive it. Studies have shown that being in a group of similar women can increase their feelings of value and lead to experiences of 'inclusion, co-operation, and mutuality' (Herman 2018, pp.166–167). Importantly, the resultant feelings of acceptance and belonging felt by the women in the group as they explored their body image issues may also have contributed to an amelioration of long-held feelings of stigma and shame (Herman & Schatzow 1984).

5 Case Studies, Study Two

Metaphor, Symbolism, and Body Image

Priscilla, Cynthia, and Nancy: Metaphor and Symbolism

Within this chapter, the case studies, drawn from Study Two of Dr Trisha Crocker's PhD research project, featuring the work of Priscilla, Cynthia, and Nancy, are presented and discussed in relation to the themes of metaphor, symbolism, and body image. Priscilla and Cynthia both used metaphor and symbolism to explore body image issues around aging and the various issues it brings with it. At the time of the sessions both women were aged 52 years. The early 50s are significant as this is the age when most women experience the onset of the menopause and the various body changes, along with the psychological changes this brings. It may also be the optimum time for a 'mid-life' review of one's life so far, learning from the past in order to inform the future.

Cynthia

The three women participating on different days began with a lump or block of clay, which for Cynthia equated to a 'blank slate':

> "No. I'm, kind of, a bit stuck, actually. I'm wondering why that is. I just – maybe it's good to start – to start off with another, kind of [pause] – I want to make this perfect [laughs] perfect block, and it's not going to happen. You know, like this concrete slab, like a building block, I suppose."
>
> *Cynthia*

While she was holding the sticky clay, and feeling 'a bit stuck', Cynthia suggested that she wanted to make a 'perfect' building block but reflected that "it's not going to happen", suggesting she was anxious about making mistakes initially. However, she recognised that being involved in the creative process, smoothing and scraping the clay, meant that she was able to talk about what she was doing . . . reflecting on the process:

> "[It's] rather nice because I'm, sort of, talking, but I'm not really thinking about what I'm making. I suppose I can't think – I suppose I can't do – I suppose it's helping me talk."
>
> *Cynthia*

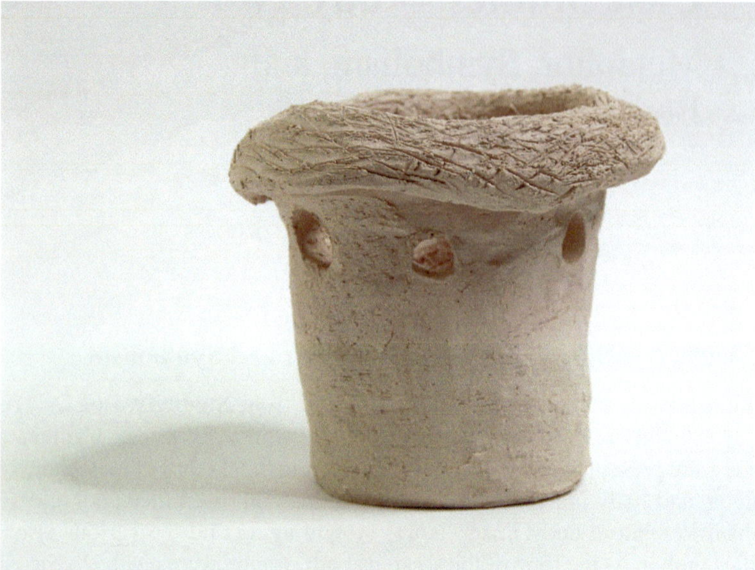

Figure 33 Sculpture No. 3 by *Cynthia*.
"The Container Outside."

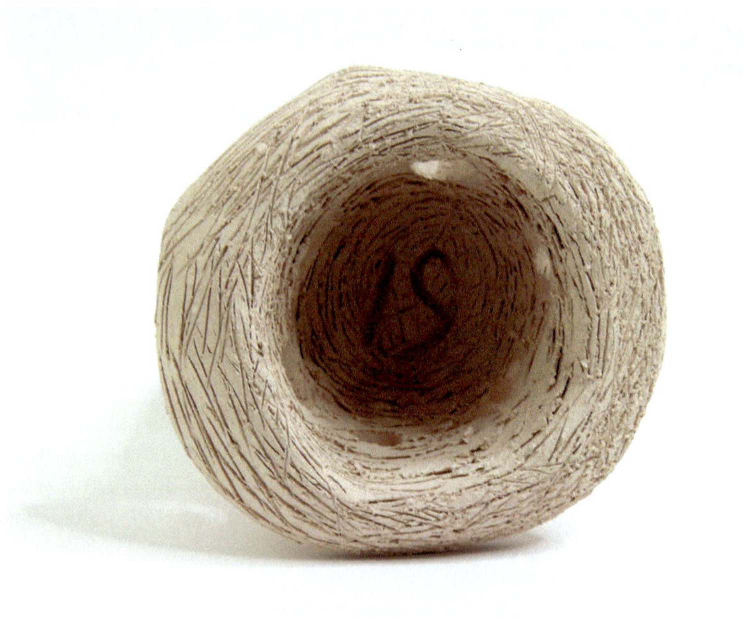

Figure 34 Sculpture No. 3 by *Cynthia*.
"The Container Inside."

Attempting to make sense of her emotions while talking with the clay in her hands Cynthia had as yet not begun to make anything with it. She had mentioned she felt a bit stuck and didn't know where to begin.

Cynthia's statement that she was seeking change and for new things to take place in her life seemed significant. With the block of clay in her hands, Cynthia seemed to be seeking inspiration, saying it reminded her of going on a journey. The thoughts that Cynthia expressed suggested that she was thinking back to times and places in her life which had significant meaning. Reviewing her past seemed to be a precursor for Cynthia beginning to make sense of what she wanted her future to be, and think about a new start. Cynthia also talked about her image (see Figures 33 & 34) as representing a container that symbolised her internal feelings, and talked of placing a candle in the container.

> "And I'm thinking about the candle now. I'm thinking about lighting the candle in there and thinking about that, too . . ."
>
> *Cynthia*

> "And the scratches are really – actually, the more – I really – they brought out lots of thoughts and feelings for me, and I was using this very sharp tool for the clay, to make these marks."
>
> *Cynthia*

Cynthia made the cuts and scratches mostly inside the clay vessel, but it appeared as though they were pouring out like a liquid. The incisions became deeper and deeper as Cynthia worked on her image with the sharp tool, *and* which suggested pain and anger and self-harm. Cynthia proceeded to take the other clay body image sculptures she had made off the shelf and looked at the three together.

> "Oh, yeah. They're all, sort of, related. Well, the two [container-like ones] sort of . . . but not the owl [. . .] woman-owl thing."
>
> *Cynthia*

Cynthia talks here about how she sees two of her three body image sculptures (see Figures 27 on p.80, 32 on p.85 & 33) as related to each other; however, they all seem related to her journey. These were the "mushroom", which speaks of coming out of the darkness and the group said appeared to represent female genitalia, "the Owl woman in the baggy trousers" which represented the aging body and death, and the last "open vessel" on which Cynthia inscribed her pain, and then created "portholes" through which she could see her "enemies" and through which she could be seen "a little bit". Cynthia finally decided that a candle could be placed within the "open vessel", to let in the light, suggesting Cynthia finally considered herself worthy of 'being seen'.

Using metaphor and symbolism as a way to focus on the psychological elements of body image rather than the physiological aspects, encouraged reflection in both the group sessions and the individual sessions. As both types of sessions were undirected, in that the participants were able to produce any image that reflected their body image, they were not restricted to creating a realistic image. This meant that Cynthia was able to begin her clay sculpture in a creative abstract way without any preconceptions, developing this into something that reflected her body image.

> ". . . look, because I don't – I'm only just starting to shape. I've just started realising I actually have the power to shape who I am."
>
> *Cynthia*

This was an important breakthrough for Cynthia, realising she had the 'power' to shape who she was, both physically by creating an image, and through the use of metaphor and symbolism.

The cuts Cynthia made into her clay sculpture (see Figure 34 on p.92), were indicative of anger and self-harm; however, Cynthia talked about the root cause of this:

> "Ugly, ugly, yeah. My – yeah, I'm starting to – it's about the ugly parts of myself."
>
> *Cynthia*

Exploring the cuts into the clay she had made, Cynthia suggested that they were about the 'ugly' parts of herself. Although she used the word 'ugly' Cynthia seemed to be referring to both internal and external elements of herself.

> "Letting them show more, or not feeling I've got to hide them, either my physical thing – either physical things from the outside, or my anger, for instance, because I think that's something that I've hidden."
>
> *Cynthia*

Cynthia spoke about how she was letting the marks relating to anger and ugliness show more as she scratched the top as well as the inside of her sculpture. Using metaphor and symbolism when producing her body image may have been a safer option for Cynthia, as this can be seen as less revealing than producing a realistic image of herself, which would be painful for herself to see.

Cynthia did not stop working on her sculpture (see Figure 33 on p.92) at this point, but discussed the further additions she had made and was making:

> "Well, I've made these little – the little portholes round the edge, and I – they're like, kind of, a castle, like a fortress, you know, when it has the little lookout place so you can see the enemy coming. But also, they can look in and see you, so it's both ways. And you can be seen a little bit. And the other – the other thing I thought about was, like, a tea light.

It actually reminds me a bit of a tea light holder and how I'd like to put a candle inside it, because I feel that – I feel my mood – I feel a lot happier in myself, and I think it's a happy – when I seek that place now, it's more of a happier solitude than it was before."

Cynthia

Art Therapist/Researcher Reflective Diary

I wondered who 'the enemy' was that she might see from inside the portholes. This might have been a theme to pursue further with Cynthia had the time restrictions on the study allowed.

For Cynthia, her abstract sculpture (see Figure 33 on p.92) enabled a narrative to be built around it, full of metaphor and symbolism. One that began with angry cathartic cuts into the clay form, and an admission that she 'hates' her body image, which then transitioned into a protective space, a fortress or castle that she could 'withdraw to', a space with 'portholes' through which 'enemies' could be seen and through which she could also be seen 'a little bit'. Finally, the sculpture becomes a space to hold and display *light*, by placing a candle within it, perhaps signalling a new beginning, and a recognition that her body can be a positive thing filled with light, if she is ready to 'look at herself' and *accept* who she is.

The following extract seems to indicate that Cynthia was finding a way, through the clay sculptures, to rationalise her progression as she identifies that the metaphor and symbolism used to describe her sculpture has gone from a "fortress" to a "dead kind of thing" to something "more alive".

"And also, it's a protection [. . .] it's protecting my own space, as well as being – or maybe instead of being a place to withdraw, it's actually a positive space where you can withdraw to or I can withdraw to when I want to, and bring in the things that I want to have there, rather than feel I *should* . . . or, you know, that kind of stuff. But it's also to do with nature. I think these marks, they make it – that they make this feel more like an organic thing, and it's something more alive, and something living rather than a, sort of, very smooth, dead kind of thing. This one's more flowing and this is more living. The scratchy bit is more, more of a living thing, I think, more alive, so – and that's how I do feel."

Cynthia

Here Cynthia is referring to her sculpture from Study One (see Figure 32 on p.85) which she had referred to as the "mushroom shape", describing it as a "very, smooth, dead kind of thing". The group had also reflected on the sculpture's similarity in shape to female genitalia, suggesting it was a metaphor perhaps related to sex and aging, and the loss of her relationship.

The metaphor of a 'mushroom/vagina' is an interesting one as mushrooms are actually the visible sex organs of the microbe Fungi that produces them. Mushrooms also emerge from the *darkness* into the *light*, and have been associated with mythology and magic, e.g. in fairy-tale and fantasy.

Art Therapist/Researcher Reflective Diary

I reflected that 'mushroom' as a metaphor features in one of Sylvia Plath's poems entitled *Mushrooms* (1959). The text highlights similarities with women's body image issues around aging and invisibility where Plath says "Nobody sees us [. . .]" and also on dieting and being slim . . . "We diet on water, on crumbs of shadow bland-mannered, asking little or nothing. So many of us!" (from Sylvia Plath's *Mushrooms*, 1959.

> "Oh, yeah, the mushroom. It started looking like a mushroom, initially, and I was thinking about how I have been – I feel like I have been in the dark and hiding, like a mushroom. Mushrooms are, sort of – that's how they grow, in the dark, don't they? And then, I – it reminded me of when my son said to me several years ago, "Mum, stop hiding".
>
> *Cynthia*

Bringing the 'light' into her sculpture was therefore a significant thing for Cynthia. Perhaps it indicated that Cynthia was 'seeing the light' for the first time. She realised the truth of her son's words and appeared ready to move forward and emerge from the dark. Demonstrating how even in a few sessions of using clay to explore body image, Cynthia was able to see what was happening for her and for many other women, in comparing her body to the unattainable cultural ideals regarding female body image, and to begin to develop self-compassion and understanding.

Cynthia described the mushroom shape and circular piece inside the mushroom/vagina as exposing her internal discomfort and unhappiness. However, through the use of clay, Cynthia was able to create a physical object that represented her experience of embodiment, rather than a realistic image of herself, meaning she was able to create a narrative around this, full of metaphor and symbolism. Having a three-dimensional object meant that Cynthia was able to view it from all angles, and literally stand back and view it more objectively, gaining insight into her issues, recognising the defences she has put up around herself, and finally her objective to fill the space created with light and positivity.

Art Therapist/Researcher Reflective Diary

During the discussion I had the feeling of being on a roller coaster as I listened to Cynthia, with her emotions going up and down, providing excitement and confusion in quick succession. I sensed that Cynthia was feeling as if she had emerged from the container, as she addressed the scratches that she had made (see Figure 33 on p.92).

> "It's pain. It's pain. It's something about pain, as well."
>
> *Cynthia*

Cynthia continued to speak of this new sculpture (Figure 33 on p.92) and suggested that 'the pain' might be about feeling hurt, and the shame and resulting pain of all women who do not feel 'good enough', or who are judged by their body shape or weight, rather than for *who* or *what* they are.

Cynthia said that the scratches incised into the clay were 'more organic', which suggested a sense of growth and movement, in contrast to her previous 'mushroom' piece that she described as 'dead', and 'stuck'. She also referred to the new sculpture as an 'open vessel', a place that lets in *light* and the *living*, as such it seemed to indicate feelings of *hope*.

> "[. . .] There are a lot, rather a lot. But it's, like, not just me. [. . .] The more I get to know people and the more I'm sharing with people, either patients or friends, I'm letting in other people – or I'm listening more to other people's things that aren't so nice."
>
> *Cynthia*

This suggests that Cynthia was beginning to open up about her feelings, sharing more of herself with friends and colleagues, and listening to the issues they also experience. Recognising that most women have body image issues and fears of not being 'good enough' meant letting go of the idea that other women were 'perfect', and beginning to accept that most women have body image issues similar to hers. This feeling of solidarity with other women has been shown to help ameliorate painful feelings of isolation and loss, or fear of being ostracised for not fitting in to the unrealistic ideals created by society.

Through creating abstract and semi-abstract sculptures (see Figures 27 on p.80, 32 on p.85 & 33 on p.92), Cynthia was able to include metaphor and symbolism to safely explore her pain and anger. As discussed in Chapter 2, feelings of shame around body image can cause extensive feelings of pain and suffering for women, and that it is in developing self-compassion that women are able to ameliorate feelings of body-shame.

Nancy

Un-met expectations and assumptions about how she believed her life should be was a theme that occurred frequently for Nancy.

> "I think that was a big turning point for me, you know, sort of, ending a relationship at an age where I thought I should be – well – when everyone else was getting married and having children, and at a point when I assumed that that would be happening for me."
>
> *Nancy*

However, Nancy talks philosophically and suggests that *acceptance* is her only way forward:

> ". . . this is maybe just how it is and I need to, kind of, just get on with it and accept the consequences . . ."
>
> *Nancy.*

Art Therapist/Researcher Reflective Diary

I reflected that deciding to 'accept the consequences' suggested that Nancy could not see herself doing anything other than that. She appeared to be unable to make changes, and found it easier to just accept her circumstances and not to try changing them.

> "Because I have all of those expectations of myself to . . . kind of . . . manage and do things . . . but I just haven't *wanted* to do it."
>
> *Nancy*

This suggests a feeling of apathy, a lack of motivation, or even a sense of 'lacking' in herself, . . . inferring that she is unable to "manage and do things".

However, Nancy does recognise that her expectations need to change in order to move forward. When Nancy refers to her need to "accept the consequences", it seems an acknowledgement that moving forward, and change, will bring about further issues for her to face, but that she is preparing herself to do this.

> "I am not a proper woman. I can't do two things at once. But I think that's it. I just – I felt really – I have felt really overwhelmed since January, of feeling really [. . .] and I just, kind of, just got on with it, and I think I'm starting to see little bits, like . . . not doing the washing up and stuff like that. It was maybe a signal that just everything feels a bit too much."
>
> *Nancy*

> **Art Therapist/Researcher Reflective Diary**
>
> Nancy suggests that she is not a 'proper woman', in that she is unable to multi-task. I wonder where her ideas of a 'proper woman' came from, perhaps her Mother?

Nancy suggested that she thought a "proper woman" would be able to cope and not feel overwhelmed by the changes and issues in her life. Nancy's admission that she doesn't see herself as a 'proper woman' implies she was unable to meet her own expectations, and was therefore a disappointment to herself. This belief that she was a 'failure' as a woman added a further complexity to Nancy's negative body image.

Priscilla

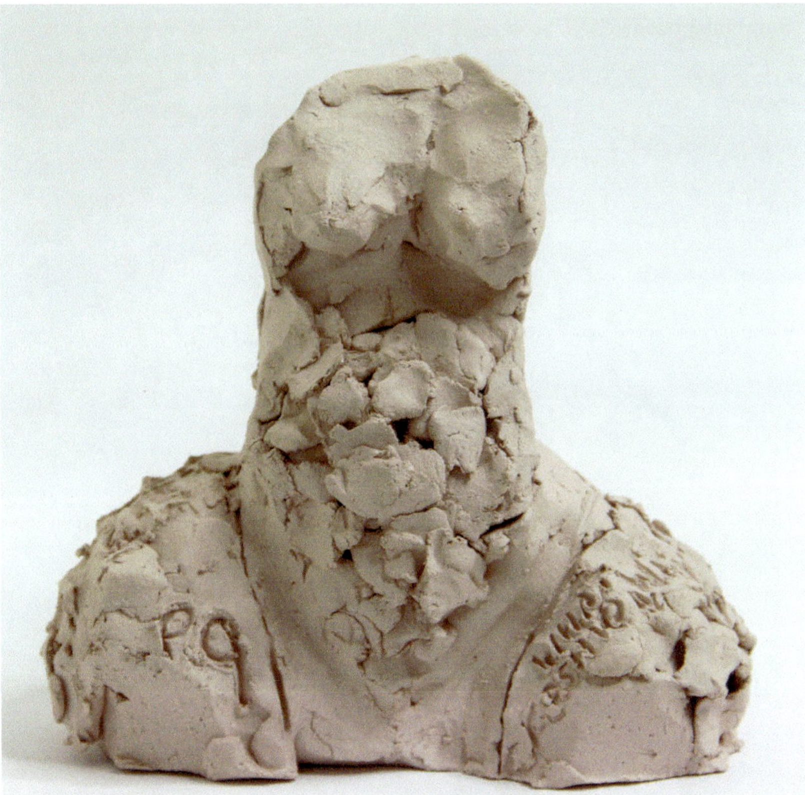

Figure 35 Sculpture No. 2 by *Priscilla.*
"Torso with Large Hips and Angry Words."

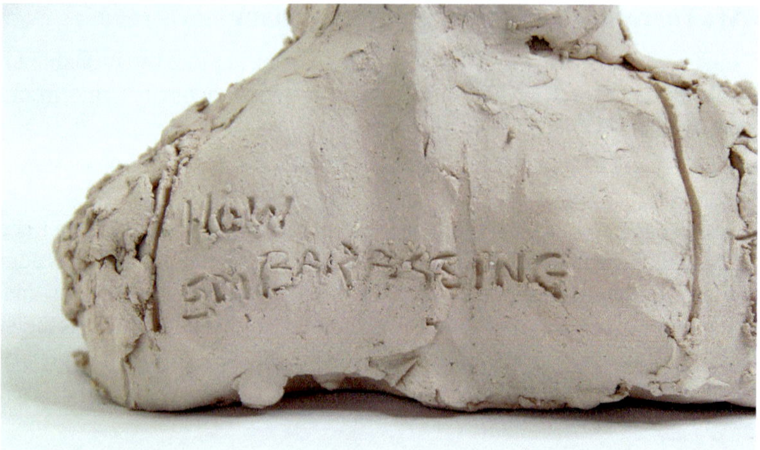

Figure 36 Sculpture No. 1 by *Priscilla.*
"How Embarrassing."

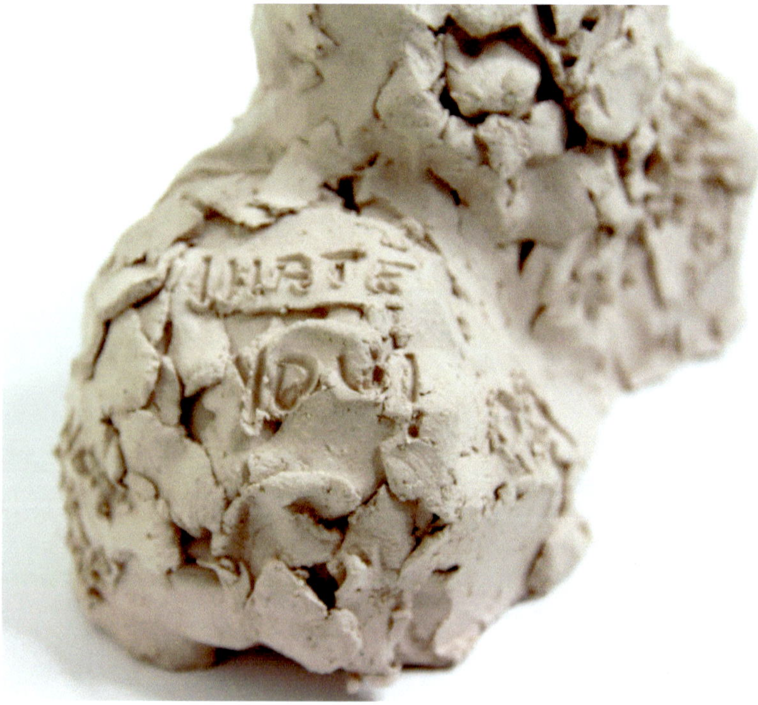

Figure 37 Sculpture No. 1 by *Priscilla.*
"I Hate You."

Priscilla's first sculpture created during Study One was a "torso with large hips and angry words" (see Figure 35 on p.99) such as "how embarrassing" (see Figure 36) and "I hate you" (see Figure 37) inscribed deeply with a sharp tool into different body parts on the sculpture. Priscilla initially worked with the clay without speaking and appeared visibly angry as she stabbed and scratched the words into her sculpture, however this led to a lengthy process of personal reflection, raising body image issues that Priscilla claimed she had rarely voiced before.

The completed sculpture depicted a shape with large hips and an upright torso with small breasts. Priscilla said that the erect nature of the sculpture reflected how she thought others saw her, i.e. confident and outspoken.

Art Therapist/Researcher Reflective Diary

I reflected that this contrasted with how Priscilla presented during the discussions, as she often had to be prompted to engage in the conversations. I was also struck by the image's similarity to a phallic symbol; however this was not recognised or brought up by the group, and therefore not discussed.

Inscribing angry words into her body image with a sharp clay tool, so that they would not be hidden or difficult to decipher, suggests that Priscilla had decided to express feelings that she had previously kept hidden, wanting the words to be read by the other members of the group.

In the Study One group discussions Priscilla had challenged any positive remarks from fellow participants about accepting her size. Priscilla even became angry and suggested that the other women were not being open or saying what they really felt. It seemed that Priscilla's defences would not allow any compassion or positivity to reach her.

Priscilla begins to unpick some of her body image issues when she says:

> "It's a half-baked . . . well, I don't know . . . I think [pause] . . . it's really rather how you *see* yourself, isn't it? It's whether you *see* yourself or whether you *are* yourself."
>
> *Priscilla*

This suggests that Priscilla is unable to *see* herself and *be* herself at the same time, and may be dissociating from her body image, perhaps meaning that she is unable to see herself as others see her.

Art Therapist/Researcher Reflective Diary

I wondered if Priscilla's body image was in some way distorted by previous pain/shame around body image. It seemed that Priscilla's body image was 'off limits', making it very difficult for her to create and view her body image.

Some of this was explained when Priscilla admitted that she couldn't even look at herself in a mirror:

> "It's still . . . I still feel uncomfortable. [. . .] Yeah . . . I don't look at myself in the mirror."
>
> *Priscilla*

'Being seen' by the self or others was clearly a big issue for Priscilla, and brought up significant fear, shame and pain.

Priscilla talks metaphorically about her propensity to 'live' in her head, and how this means that she is unable to 'see' herself:

> "And if you *are* yourself, you don't *see* your head, but if you *see* yourself, you *see* your head."
>
> *Priscilla*

The propensity for Priscilla to dissociate from or ignore her body meant she had no option but to 'live' in her head. This could be seen as an impassive stance, in which she sought to manage her feelings (i.e. her embodiment) by 'being in her head', i.e. *thinking* rather than *feeling*. Priscilla attempted to develop an objective *logic* to describe her body image issues, as the pain of 'experiencing' or 'embodying' the issues seemed too great.

Priscilla used metaphoric language to explain a coping mechanism she'd developed previously to avoid feeling shame and pain, meaning that she was now unable to look at herself without experiencing strong emotions that had been hidden or buried for a long time.

Art Therapist/Researcher Reflective Diary

I reflected that the emotions behind Priscilla's discussion were 'held' mainly when in contact with others, and that when Priscilla was alone, she may have found it more difficult to keep them at bay.

It seemed that Priscilla saw herself as someone who used rational, intellectual reasoning, rather than being in touch with her emotions. Priscilla found it difficult to focus on the physical visual aspects of body image, preferring to remain 'in her head' and concentrate on the internal psychological processing, and seemed to have developed a coping strategy of ignoring her physical self to avoid cognitive dissonance (Festinger 1962). Cognitive dissonance is about having two conflicting beliefs at the same time (ibid.), the conflict here being a miss-match between the *fantasy* and *reality* regarding Priscilla's body image. This equated to Priscilla managing to 'be' herself, by dissociating from a body that she did not accept as part of who she was. Consequently, looking in the mirror would mean the shattering of Priscilla's 'fantasy' body image.

Cynthia

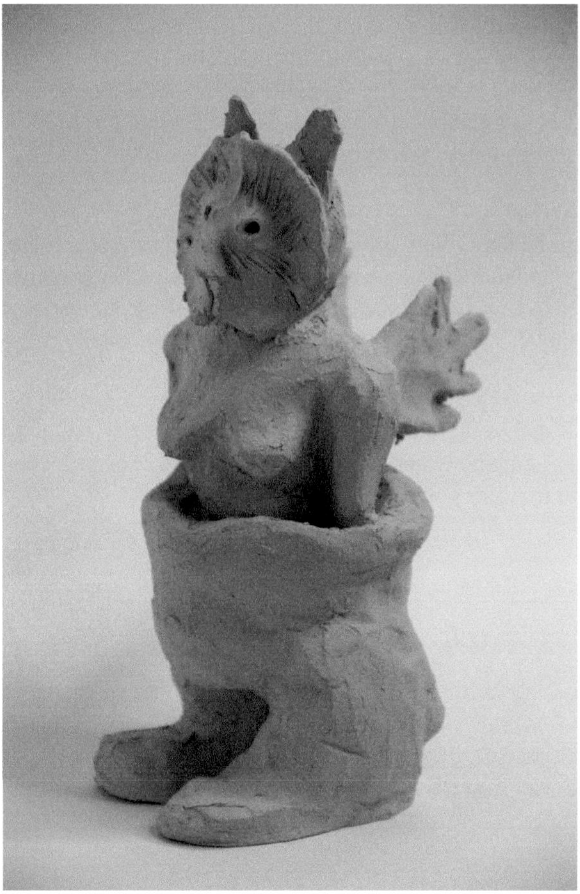

Figure 38 (see also Figures 27 & 28 on p.80) Sculpture No. 1 by *Cynthia*. "The Owl in Baggy Trousers."

Cynthia's first sculpture, which she sometimes referred to as "The Owl in Baggy Trousers" (see Figure 38 on p.103, and also Figures 27 & 28 on p.80), was created during Study One but was also referred to in the dialogue of Study Two as Cynthia reflected on her aging body. Cynthia referred to her age often during the sessions, sometimes saying that she felt older than her 52 years, having to remind herself that she could still do things like take exercise:

> "And I Googled, Am I too old to start running? . . . And I'm thinking, I'm only 52, actually."
>
> *Cynthia*

Cynthia's remarks about her age appeared to be all-consuming and defining of her body image as she reflected on the losses in her life:

> "I feel quite sad though, at the same time, because I feel I've – there's a lot of loss. And I feel – I think that the feeling is . . . *I've missed the bus* [laughter]. Just a waste, and I do feel sad about that, because of – I know there's no point in saying . . . in hindsight . . . 'Oh, if only,' – but I do fantasise quite a lot about if I had felt like this when I was 30, maybe. But, you know, it's crazy, you know."
>
> *Cynthia*

Cynthia spoke about how her aging body had made her more conscious of her mortality, and that this new awareness had enabled her to consider how she really wanted to live as best she could for herself, something she describes as a 'positive' move:

> "And that's very much on my mind, and me, really, at the moment. And I think it makes me more conscious of my mortality . . . and how I must live – my aging body and how I really want to live as best I can for myself now, and it's very positive."
>
> *Cynthia*

Art Therapist/Researcher Reflective Diary

I wondered about the seeming contradiction in using the words 'mortality' and 'aging' versus 'living' and 'positive' and wondered if this showed a sense of uncertainty and inner conflict, as Cynthia looked for a realistic way forward with her life.

What came through strongly when listening to Cynthia was a growing recognition that she needed to change her attitudes and beliefs about her body image in order to move forward with her life in a positive way. It seemed that Cynthia felt being 52 years of age was a wakeup call for her, acknowledging that time had been wasted with decades of feeling bad about her body image. Cynthia also reflected on the recent end of her marriage:

> ". . . with both of that, with the ending of a relationship and with the fact I'm [still] living with this person, with a failed relationship, that feels like an ending and a death, too."
>
> *Cynthia*

Cynthia's body image sculpture, "The Owl in Baggy Trousers" (see Figure 38 on p.103), takes on a new significance considering the symbolic meaning of the 'owl' which has traditionally been seen as a symbol of wisdom, but also of death (particularly in Native American mythology). This suggests that within her body image sculpture Cynthia was reflecting upon both aging and death, but also the new 'wisdom' she was discovering through the process. Significant endings often provoke a period of reflection and re-evaluation of one's life, its direction, and its meaning, and can be likened to holding up a mirror to one's self, just as creating her body image in clay was like holding up a mirror for Cynthia.

Priscilla

Priscilla discussed cutting away at her second clay sculpture (see Figure 39) in order to shape it more to her liking, however she became concerned that if

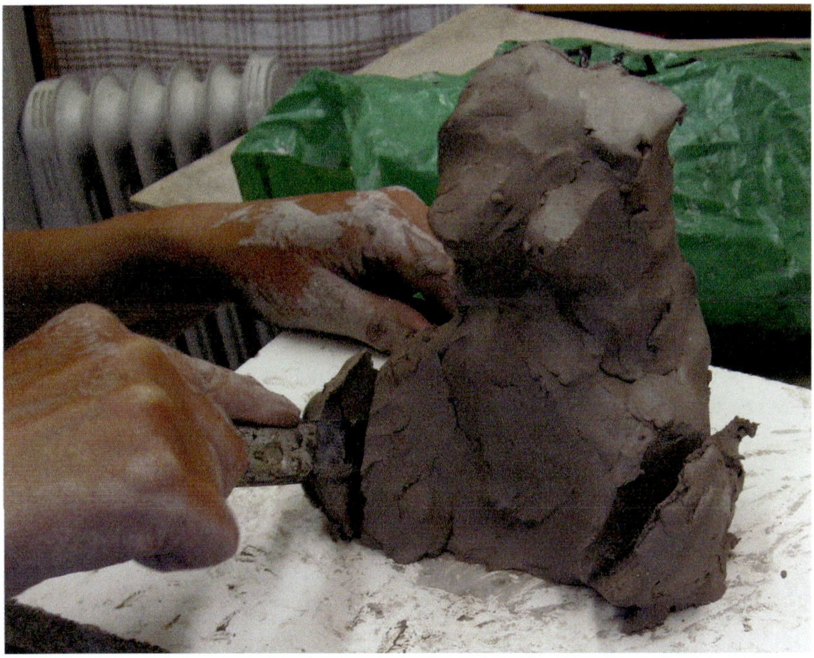

Figure 39 Sculpture No. 2 by *Priscilla.*
"Cutting Away."

she did, she would not *recognise* herself. After deliberating for a while Priscilla decided to 'have a go' and cut off some clay to change the body image sculpture she was making of herself.

> **Art Therapist/Researcher Reflective Diary**
>
> I wondered if this meant Priscilla was not ready to change the way she perceived herself, because that would mean changing her long-held beliefs about her body.

> "Well, you'd just have a smaller – you'd just have a, sort of, a smaller section of bottom and hip. I mean it literally is eight inches. So, I'd be quite [laughs] – you know had I done my legs [pause]? But I can't actually work out the curve [laughs]. Well, I can have a go. I'm not sure how I feel about disconnecting myself."
>
> *Priscilla*

Priscilla's laughter perhaps suggests embarrassment at pointing out the areas of her body she was most uncomfortable with, but could also have indicated embarrassment regarding a lack of skills in sculpting. However, 'having a go' meant that Priscilla was willing to continue playing with the clay, cutting and moving the clay on the sculpture, and therefore consider changing her body image.

> "Well, that's how I think of myself more, I suppose, if I don't see any pictures. Just, kind of – yeah, I don't need to look perfect. That would be really nice. There you go. More of a waist, a bit less of a tummy [. . .]."
>
> *Priscilla*

Priscilla moves to a more balanced position on her body image as she recognises "I don't need to look perfect." Priscilla pointed out that the buttocks on her sculpture were not shaped, and was surprised that it was not 'perfection' that she was looking for.

> "Yeah. That's alright, excellent. Yes, well, there you are [pause]. And I suppose my reluctance to chop bits off and, you know, reject them . . ."
>
> *Priscilla*

Priscilla used the words 'alright' and 'excellent' to describe her body image sculpture intimating her positive perception of it after she had modified it, whilst also admitting that it was more representative of her actual body image.

In her first body image sculpture (see Figures 17 on p.69, 18 & 19 on p.70) Priscilla explored her large hips, and her anger at having to live with them was inscribed upon it. Priscilla's second image (see Figure 39 on p.105) allowed her to focus on her body from a more positive and realistic viewpoint. This demonstrates the power of clay work as a tool to help women to physically explore their body image within a therapeutic environment.

Priscilla's written replies on her Study Two questionnaire completed at the end of the session, substantiate the power of clay work, and demonstrate how working with clay helps the creator explore their personal body image issues, giving them the opportunity to recognise, discuss, and move away from internalised shame through modifying or revisioning their body image.

6 Case Studies, Study Two

Mothers' and Others' Influence on Body Image

Priscilla, Cynthia, and Nancy: Mothers' and Others' Influence

Within this chapter the case studies, drawn from Study Two of Dr Trisha Crocker's PhD research project, featuring the work of Priscilla, Cynthia, and Nancy, are presented and discussed in relation to the themes of mothers' and others' influence on body image. All three women in study two spoke of the substantial influence their mothers had on the way they have viewed their bodies throughout life. It was also one of the themes discussed by most of the participants in Study One;

Here Helena talks about her 9-year-old daughter and the effect her own words as a mother might have on her:

> "You know she will say . . . oh, am I fat? Do I look thin? Do I look fat? I know that there's like, a little joke where I've always like, said to her, 'Oh, I hope you don't have, I hope you have legs like daddy, you don't have legs, thunder thighs like mummy.' You know. And then I forget that I'm saying it, but I wonder if a comment like that would actually stay with her, you know."
>
> *Helena*

The impact of the critical mother on a daughter's body image was therefore one of the key themes that arose during the study, and one of the most significant.

Priscilla

Priscilla's mother emerged as someone who had often reminded Priscilla of all her perceived body issues, and although it appeared that her mother did not intentionally criticise her to cause shame and hurt, Priscilla's already negative body image seemed to have been impaired to a high degree by the things her mother said. Priscilla's ability to clearly recall hurtful things that her mother had said to her in childhood is an indication that they made a significant impact (Berntsen 2001).

It seemed from Priscilla's dialogue that her mother was also uncomfortable with her own body, this discomfort was then passed down to Priscilla. Priscilla's mother compared her body shape to Priscilla's, suggesting that because Priscilla was taller, she would be able to 'hide' the defects:

> "I've had . . . you get comments, I think. My mother was always very aware of the fact that she had . . . she was the same, although much shorter. She always said, 'It's fantastic you've got such broad shoulders, you know, and you can hide it . . .'"
>
> *Priscilla*

Although Priscilla's mother may have been trying to support and reassure her daughter, inadvertently her words reinforced Priscilla's body image issues.

Art Therapist/Researcher Reflective Diary

I reflected that perhaps the comments Priscilla's mother made were meant as an innocuous comment, or perhaps it was a 'passive-aggressive' attack on Priscilla's body image? Priscilla's mother may also have felt anger and shame about her own body image, and wanted Priscilla to share the *burden* of her personal dissatisfaction with her body . . . as she said to Priscilla . . . "you have broad shoulders . . ."

By suggesting that Priscilla could 'hide' her body imperfections, Priscilla's mother was implying that there was something *unacceptable* or *abnormal* about Priscilla's body, something she should be ashamed of. Also, saying that Priscilla had 'such broad shoulders' indicated that Priscilla's body was 'unfeminine' . . . perhaps adding to Priscilla's confusion and dislike of her own body. This underlines the substantial power a critical (m)other has in building or decreasing body image satisfaction in their daughters.

The idea of 'hiding' one's body continued as Priscilla talked about her mother's own dislike of showing her body, e.g. her loathing of bikinis or swimsuits:

> "And, you know, there's a similar thing about bikinis, and it's just that – maybe that over-analysis came from my mother, I don't know. She was, sort of very keen on, you know, what it looked like, but [. . .] I don't know. I mean she has a very similar shape to mine, except she's much shorter and much smaller. And, in fact, her issues are slightly worse. But, I mean, she was – she just wouldn't wear a swimming costume or stuff. [. . .] Yes, saying 'It's a shame you've got my shape', or whatever. But, even worse, predicting that I would look just like her . . ."
>
> *Priscilla*

A personal negative body image, meant that Priscilla's mother most probably passed on these negative beliefs to her daughter, and these issues may also have been historical and intergenerational, meaning that they were passed down to Priscilla through several generations. Priscilla's mother may have been attempting to find solidarity and compassion in sharing her own body image issues with her daughter, however, by suggesting that Priscilla had inherited her mother's body shape and predicting that she would 'look just like her' was counterproductive. Priscilla's distress is understandable considering that these negative comments were said by her 'mother', when 'a good enough (m)other' should provide unconditional love and support to their child.

Consequently, Priscilla developed a sense of personal *shame*, believing her body to be unacceptable, and something to be hidden from view. Priscilla's mother may also have been attempting to protect her daughter from receiving negative comments from others, by suggesting that she 'hide' her body. Also suggesting to Priscilla that there are certain clothes that she should never wear, such as swimming costumes and bikinis, may have given her an anxiety regarding shopping for clothes, something she describes as "humiliating":

> "And then, one of my grandmothers wanted to take me shopping, and of course, you know, she could try stuff on and it all fitted, and there was nothing that actually fitted me. And it was just – it's almost humiliating, actually, that sort of thing. And it's not because anybody's saying anything, but it's just that fact that nothing really fits. So, it's actually quite limiting, I suppose . . ."
>
> *Priscilla*

Being unable to 'fit into' any of the clothes available was likely to have emphasised in Priscilla's mind that she was not 'normal', that her body shape was not catered for in mainstream shops. Priscilla talks of *humiliation* and *shame*, and her detailed memory of this shopping trip from decades previously suggests it was also traumatic due to the persistence of *traumatic memories* (Berntsen 2001).

Priscilla also talks about her memory of other hurtful comments received from 'others':

> "I was going to stay with some friends, and they had a younger – she had a younger brother [pause] who said to her . . . 'Hasn't she got huge hips or thighs, or something.' And it was – he was only young, so he wasn't actually saying it in a – in any way other than observational. And so, you know, she told me . . . and so, there's a lot of that stuff that goes on . . ."
>
> *Priscilla*

The negativity Priscilla already felt about her body appeared to have been deepened by persistent memories of a young boy noticing and pointing out her 'huge hips or thighs', as if they were something shocking or amusing, or something that he had never seen before, and couldn't quite believe.

As indicated by Priscilla's discomfort whilst shopping with her grandmother, clothes shopping was a major stressor for Priscilla, as she has described her difficulty in finding any clothes to fit. Therefore, an incident when she lost a suitcase containing all her holiday clothes became her 'worst nightmare' because she was forced to go clothes shopping with an uncle:

> "I went on holiday with my uncle and his family, and my suitcase got lost. So, it was one of those, I had to buy everything, and of course, actually buying things like swimming costumes and trousers is my worst nightmare. I hate shopping, and I had to go and do that with my uncle. And it was like, oh God, that's awful . . ."
>
> *Priscilla*

Again, this underlines Priscilla's feelings of body-shame about her shape, and extreme anxiety that she would not find anything to 'fit into', causing her to feel humiliated and different. There is also a suggestion that shopping with an *uncle*, rather than an *aunt* exacerbated the issues, in that he was unlikely to give Priscilla the empathy or understanding that a fellow female may have offered.

From an evolutionary point of view, being 'different' risks being ostracised and excluded from the community, something that historically could result in abandonment and death. Therefore, the anxiety this caused Priscilla, even on an unconscious level, was likely to have been high. This underlines the substantial power 'mothers' and 'others' have in building or decreasing body image satisfaction in their daughters, and the development of an inner critic.

Priscilla described developing a survival technique regarding her body issues throughout her life as a process of 'disconnecting'; however, she had a propensity to continually 'discuss' these issues with herself, suggesting an *inability* to 'disconnect'. Priscilla also had high expectations of herself, which presented a barrier to developing acceptance:

> "It shouldn't be an issue, and I know it shouldn't . . . But at the grand old age of 52, I should be able to say, 'Actually, look, that's me. Take it or leave it.' And, in a sense, that's exactly what I do. But it still hurts, actually."
>
> *Priscilla*

Priscilla seemed to think that at the age of 52 she should be more accepting of her body image; however, as discussed in Chapter 2, research has shown that the propensity to experience body image issues does not tend to decrease with age. Emotional pain and discomfort around body image are indicative of feelings of shame, caused by comparing one's body image to the normative societal expectations of thinness as an *ideal f*or all women. Priscilla's avoidance behaviours are underlined when she says:

> "It's still . . . I still feel uncomfortable. [. . .] Yeah . . . I don't look at myself in the mirror."
>
> *Priscilla*

Nancy

Nancy suggested that her mother was a major influence on her negative body image, with her mother's words affecting the way in which Nancy viewed her own body.

> "It's funny how I think I picked up most of my mum's ways of being when I was younger, because my mum is quite judgmental. And so, I remember, being in the car and she'd see a woman who was overweight and maybe her belly was hanging out of her top or whatever, and she'd be like, 'Oh, that's just – you just don't want to see that kind of thing . . .' So, I think my judgement was always based on what my mum, sort of said."
>
> *Nancy*

Again, this suggests that being *overweight* or *unfit* is something *shameful*, something that 'you just don't want to see', and therefore something that should be *kept hidden*, and that these were judgements Nancy had assimilated from her mother. This meant that Nancy was unable to see herself or others without her mother's judgemental words coming back to haunt her.

Nancy suggested that her mother's views on what was 'acceptable' or 'unacceptable' regarding body image or exposure of the body, had largely influenced her own views, in that she found the same things objectionable. It seems likely that if Nancy's mother had not been so critical of other women's bodies, Nancy might not have inherited a similar dislike of her own body. "You just don't want to see that [. . .]", had obviously made a strong impact on Nancy's own view of what was acceptable and what was not, thereby inducing a sense of shame in Nancy when she did not meet her mother's exacting criteria.

> "And [. . .] I, kind of said, 'Oh God, if I had that, I wouldn't wear that.' And that's . . . my mum! [laughs] 'God, yeah. No, that's my mother' [laughter]. I can blame my mother for an awful lot. It's great!"
>
> *Nancy*

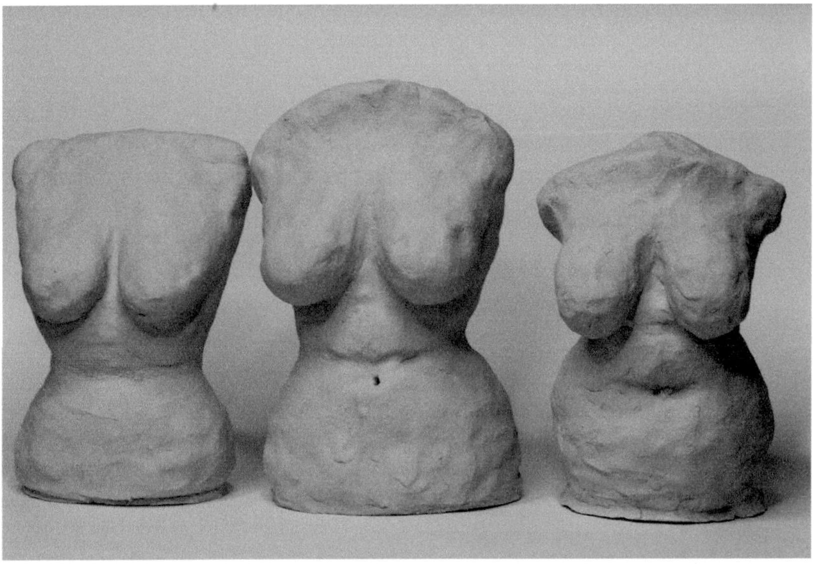

Figure 40 Sculptures Nos. 1, 2 & 3 by *Nancy.*
"For Me, It Was About Being Really Honest", or "The Three Nancys."

Art Therapist/Researcher Reflective Diary

I reflected that Nancy found it difficult to separate out her own feelings from her mother's, meaning she was unable to take responsibility for her own poor body image, but instead felt that her mother should be 'blamed' for her own feelings of body-shame and dissatisfaction.

When she worked and played with the clay, Nancy spoke freely about her body image. The words Nancy used to speak about her three sculptures (see Figure 40) implied that she felt her weight issues had always defined her and that 'pretending' had always been her coping strategy:

> "I always had a [pause] – I've always . . . you know, as I said before, I've always had an issue with my weight. Yeah, I think I've always had an issue with my weight. Yeah, I think I've always had an issue with my weight, and it was always – but I've always pretended that I didn't."
>
> *Nancy*

'Pretending' or living in a 'fantasy' as a coping strategy for body image issues does seem to be a recurring theme. It could also be seen as a process of 'covering over' her perceived body image defects. Therefore, although Nancy had an issue with her weight and appeared to have had this for much of her life, she admitted that 'pretending' 'hides' the issue.

> "And I'm more conscious of what I'm wearing, because I don't – the one thing I don't like is seeing rolls of [fat] – you know, I just always think – I always think that it's amazing when people are quite willing to show their rolls and sit there with it all, kind of, hanging out, because I just think, God, I would just be constantly trying to breathe in, or wear a baggy top. And that's it. I've been trying to wear more baggy tops so it [laughs] covers it up, and things like that."
>
> *Nancy*

Nancy's criticism of women who wear clothes that allow their 'rolls' of fat to be seen, suggests a contradiction with her admiration of women who 'just don't care' what others think. Perhaps Nancy felt that they should still cover up their bodies, whilst also not caring what others think? This may be at the root of her own issues around acceptance.

Nancy spoke as if she had more body fat than she felt was acceptable or tolerable for others to see. 'Laughing' at herself for covering her 'rolls of fat' with 'baggy tops', suggests a frustration that she was unable to comfortably reveal her body shape to others. However, 'laughing' can be used to diffuse personal embarrassment and is associated with 'openness' when interacting with others (Fink & Walker 1977, p.475).

Nancy's coping strategy regarding her body image issues had, up to this point, been to pretend that her weight was not an issue with her. The fact that she was voicing her issues whilst smoothing the clay form with her fingers suggests that the calming, sensory, soothing effects of clay work may have enabled her to finally voice these issues.

Nancy spoke of a friend she was able to confide in:

> "But she's had that ability to [. . .] grow within herself and be comfortable [pause]. So, yeah, I'm, kind of, amazed at her that she's, you know, she's just one of these people who just doesn't care. She just – you know, she just is, and it's really refreshing to be around that."
>
> *Nancy*

Nancy said her friend (who was larger than her) had a very positive attitude to her own larger shape and was comfortable in her own body. Nancy said her friend 'just doesn't care' what others think, something Nancy repeated three times, even though she admitted that she had not actually heard her friend say she 'didn't care', but that she assumed this because of how she spoke and acted.

> **Art Therapist/Researcher Reflective Diary**
>
> Nancy said she was 'amazed' at her friend's ability to 'not care' and wondered if Nancy had doubts that she herself could ever feel the same body acceptance.

Nancy's use of the word 'refreshing' suggested to me that she herself felt drained of resources in her effort to cope with her feelings around her negative body image. Nancy was 'amazed' at what she saw as her friend's body image acceptance.

Nancy continued to work on her third image while talking and comparing it with the other two. Nancy was challenging herself to cut at the clay as she talked.

> "That one's very similar, although my tummy has popped out a little bit at the bottom [laughter], which I need to put on this one [laughs]. But yeah, my tummy goes in and out as it needs to. But it does change how – it's changed how I, kind of, look in the mirror now. I, kind of, look at my body and just think, yeah, well, you know, you're a bit lumpier there, and you're a bit lumpier there, and that could be lifted and that could be tucked, and all the rest of it."
>
> *Nancy*

Nancy seemed to be challenging herself to accept the changes she saw in her body image as she worked and her laughter may have suggested embarrassment, or an effort to lighten the atmosphere. Crucially Nancy says "it's changed how I look in the mirror now", recognising that something had shifted in her mind and her way of looking at herself, something that may have influenced her decision to begin sharing her thoughts and feelings regarding her negative body image. As Nancy explained, one evening, while on a weekend course for work, she was sitting with a female colleague (who was heavier and larger in size than Nancy), when Nancy felt able to open up about her body image issues.

> "I was just sat very quietly, and it just came out. I just said, you know, "I'm really unhappy with the way I am, like my weight, the way I look, everything. I'm just really uncomfortable with it . . .". And from this point, I think doing this, doing this physical bit of coming and creating a body image [sculpture in clay] has just really helped me to – I don't know, just be honest with it, and I guess see it. [. . .] It's, kind of, like seeing something in a third person and seeing it there, reflected . . . And I came in this morning and I thought, oh God, okay, that is much bigger than the last one.

> And, you know, it was, kind of, just looking at them both. But I think the top one is absolutely gorgeous."
>
> *Nancy*

This appeared to be a turning point for Nancy, being able to refer to her own body image sculpture as 'absolutely gorgeous' and gaining the confidence to share her body image story with a female colleague. This may have increased Nancy's feelings of womanly solidarity and support around body image issues, something that she had perhaps not felt before, and something that had helped lift a metaphorical 'weight' from her shoulders:

> "Yeah, and I just started to feel better. It felt like a weight was lifted off my shoulders . . . that I had said it . . . and I was being honest."
>
> *Nancy*

Art Therapist/Researcher Reflective Diary

As this took place not long after Nancy was involved in Study One, I wondered if talking with her peers in the group discussion encouraged Nancy to be more open about her negative feelings with other women. Perhaps she had begun to realise that many other women feel a similar way about their bodies.

Cynthia

Cynthia described 'negative voices' from her childhood as being an underlying cause of the body image issues she has experienced throughout her life, in particular the voice of her mother. Cynthia used a cognitive-focused, rather than an emotion-focused, approach to understanding the discomfort she feels, and has felt historically, about her body image. It appeared that Cynthia could easily recall what had been said to her by her mother, even though the words were not necessarily intended to be hurtful or a criticism.

> ". . . there are negative voices that come from my childhood about my legs as well, from my brother, and my size from my mum, because my mum's very petite. She's five foot two, but she's a lot smaller now because she's getting older and so she's shrinking. But I was huge! I towered over her, and I look at photographs of me and her together when I was just coming into my adolescence. I'm this big . . . I should have been quite athletic, because I was quite big . . . tall for my age and quite well-built. And my mum is little, so I felt like this big, clumsy . . . and she used to call me 'you great big whatsit' and stuff like that, and it all went in . . ."
>
> *Cynthia*

Cynthia suggested that her 'petite' mother made her feel 'big' and 'clumsy' and out of place, perhaps even abnormal in size, or an 'oddity', all of which may have negatively impacted her relationship with, and the development of, a secure attachment to her mother, and vice versa.

The opinions Cynthia's mother held about other people also appeared to have had a substantial impact on Cynthia's feelings about her own body.

> "I think she, kind of, didn't like – and I know she had a thing about 'fat' people and she's a 'fattist', as she said, and she always took care of her weight. And I think I've felt that sort of feeling about me being – and it made me feel big and, sort of – and I love my food. And I was greedy, and I ate too much because I was very needy, you know."
>
> *Cynthia*

Cynthia described herself as 'greedy' and 'needy' and 'feeling big', intimating that her feelings of negative body image began early in childhood because of her mother's tendency to talk negatively about 'fat' women and the way their bodies looked, something that fed into Cynthia's insecurity around being bigger and heavier than her mother.

There was another area of long-time concern for Cynthia when she spoke about her 'neediness'. This was addressed for the first time in Study Two, when Cynthia spoke at length about being sexually abused as a child by a neighbour. The abuse went unknown and unspoken of into her adulthood, thereby perhaps demonstrating a lack of protection by her (m)other or other care givers. Cynthia said that it wasn't until she'd had her own children that she addressed the issue with her family.

Priscilla

Making comparisons of their own body image to that of other women, was also a theme mentioned by both Priscilla and Nancy in their dialogues. They discussed the belief that their bodies were 'not good enough' by comparing them negatively to others. Nancy talked about a friend who (despite being 'larger' than Priscilla) felt 'at home' in her own body, something that Nancy said she was unable to feel. Priscilla talked about her own desire to look as good in certain clothing as others did, demonstrating that both Nancy and Priscilla were affected by their critical selves, with their dialogues revealing how they both found their body image lacking.

Priscilla spoke about how finding clothing to fit her body shape, such as jeans and bikinis, was a distinct issue for her, and the coping mechanisms she employed:

> "But in my head, if I don't have to look in a mirror, I can look perfectly normal, which means that I don't look stupid wearing a bikini, and I can

go into a shop and buy a pair of jeans or whatever, and everything fits. Whereas, my entire life, it's almost impossible to buy trousers that look alright . . . It's . . . and a bikini just doesn't work."

Priscilla

Priscilla's frustration at not being able to find clothes, including jeans, that fitted her shape, presented a challenge that she had battled with throughout her teenage years and adult life. Priscilla thought she would be able to accept her body shape through being *rational* about it; however, it seems feelings of strong discontent with her shape affected her ability to do this as Priscilla talked about feeling uncomfortable in her own skin, and dissociating from, or denying, her body by never looking in the mirror. Priscilla's negative body image even went as far as self-hatred, inscribing "I hate You" on her sculpture's hips (see Figure 37 on p.100).

There was an implication of confusion around that which Priscilla had grown to 'accept' yet 'hate' and what she considered her body shape to be. The making of a second image with clay (see Figure 39 on p.105) enabled Priscilla to change those areas of her body image that she recognised were exaggerated in her first image. Working with the clay, Priscilla knew she could control her

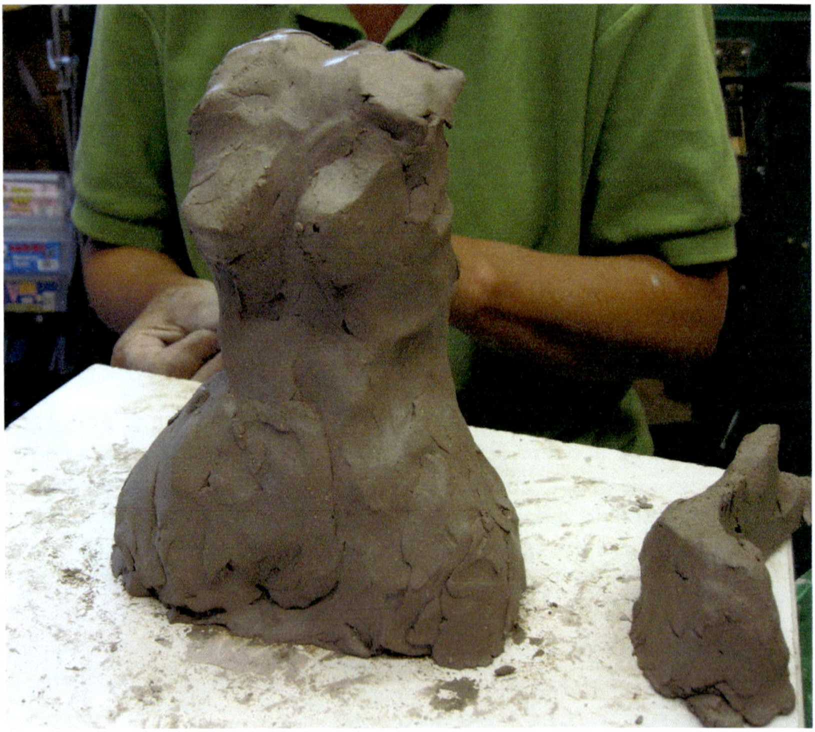

Figure 41 Sculpture No. 2 by *Priscilla.*
"Sticking It Back On."

second sculpture to her liking and perhaps as she eventually agreed, could be one that she saw as more realistic. Priscilla cut pieces of clay from the lower half of her new clay image and then she wanted to stick them back on (see Figure 41).

It seemed therefore that although Priscilla professed to 'hate' her large hips, she was having difficulty changing them.

> "But I think the only way that I can carry on is by – or have done it – is just by disconnecting completely."
>
> *Priscilla*

Realising she wanted her sculpture to represent a realistic image of herself, Priscilla laughed at the paradox she encountered.

> "I know, because, well, I didn't like seeing bits of me cut off, because I mean, I did think about, you know, liposuction and all that, and I just thought, no, I'm not doing any of that. That's just silly. And part of me goes, well, actually, that's just how – that's how God intended it, and that's just how it is. And if there weren't all these other people around . . ."
>
> *Priscilla*

Cutting large sections of clay off the hips on her sculpture was challenging to Priscilla, despite often imagining what she would look like if she could remove the parts of her body she was dissatisfied with.

Art Therapist/Researcher Reflective Diary

I reflected that there was a lot of hesitation and thought in Priscilla's movements, stopping and starting, as she cut away at the clay and then stuck it back on, as well as trying to reason that 'God intended' her shape, thereby suggesting that she *should* accept it.

When Priscilla spoke about having dismissed liposuction as 'silly', rationalising that her body was something that 'God intended', this may indicate that she was trying to be more realistic and accepting of her body image. Relating this to her work with the clay, Priscilla tried to make sense of her feelings, and the ambiguity she felt about 'seeing bits of me cut off'. What is evident is that Priscilla's ongoing battle between reality and fantasy was being played out within the clay-making session, bringing this into the light so that Priscilla could see what had been going on for her over the years. However, Priscilla seemed to be trying to deal with that internal dilemma, stating that 'part' of her felt 'that's just how it is', implying she was beginning to recognise the importance of being satisfied with what she had.

This internal conflict seemed to give rise to a sense of helplessness and the inability to effect any changes. Although Priscilla stated that she "didn't like seeing parts of me cut off" she still continued crafting her sculpture saying, "and if there weren't all these other people around . . .," implying that it was the views of others that fuelled her feelings of dissatisfaction with her body. However, Priscilla also contradicted herself, stating that it was not the views of others, but her own longstanding negative views when comparing herself to others that were difficult for her to accept.

However, as she worked on her sculpture, a change in her self-perception seemed to take place, suggesting Priscilla was able to identify with and accept the body image she was creating:

> "Yeah. I mean I don't particularly want to be anything other than that. There you go."
>
> *Priscilla*

Art Therapist/Researcher Reflective Diary

I reflected that when Priscilla said these words it was as if a light had been turned on; with both the body image sculpture and her words indicating that a fundamental sense of change and acceptance had occurred.

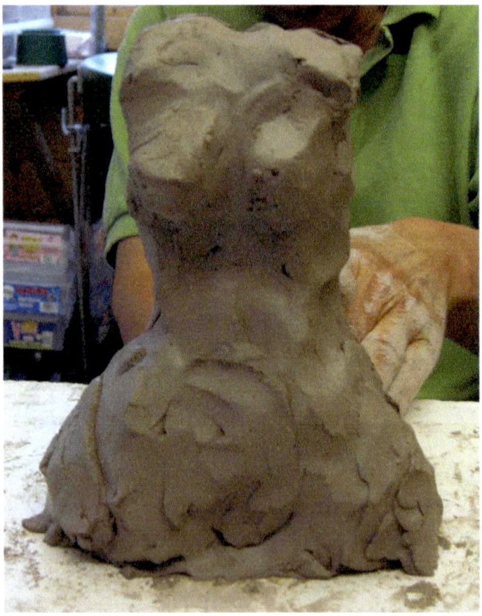

Figure 42 Sculpture No. 2 by *Priscilla.*
"That's Just How It Is."

Priscilla's final body image sculpture (see Figure 42) was clearly more realistic and balanced, yet still confirmed that her larger hips were still a part of her. Priscilla justified this change in attitude by acknowledging the 'womanliness' of her image:

> "It is a woman's body, I suppose. And maybe what's happened, is actually, it's been easier as I've grown older to have a woman's body. It's – you know, it's not really . . . a girly body . . ."
>
> *Priscilla*

This suggests that Priscilla was acknowledging that she had 'grown into' or 'matured into' her body, that perhaps it was OK to have wider hips as an 'older woman'.

Although Priscilla stated that she did not compare herself to others because it was a painful experience, she often talked of making comparisons between what others wore and what she herself was able to wear. The contradiction of not wanting to compare, yet comparing, is evident throughout the following dialogue.

> "And I don't know, I don't like looking around at what other people are wearing because I'd find it very hard to wear the same sorts of things. But in my – so, in my head, if I don't think about it, I can look like that."
>
> *Priscilla*

Making comparisons to others was something Priscilla tried to avoid, suggesting that avoidance was part of her coping strategy regarding her poor body image.

> "But I do actually sometimes feel . . . suicidal is too strong a word . . . but I do actually feel quite desperate sometimes, when I see people just . . . sort of . . . walking around wearing clothes that actually look really good, and knowing that I couldn't look like that."
>
> *Priscilla*

Undermining her body image by comparing herself to others made Priscilla feel *desperate* and the use of the word 'suicide' was disturbing, even though she said it was 'too strong a word'; however, being unable to wear the clothes that others could wear with ease, indicates feelings of 'lack of belonging' to womanhood. What women wear and how they 'dress' their bodies can be seen as part of their self-identities, therefore, part of Priscilla's self-identity was curtailed or missing because she was unable to dress or look the way she wished.

Priscilla says that, instead of feeling her pain around these issues, she prefers to 'live in her head', or in a fantasy, where she is able to wear what she pleases. As Priscilla avoids looking at herself in the mirror, this fantasy is perpetuated, despite Priscilla being aware that she does this to avoid feeling the shame/pain that a recognition of reality brings.

Priscilla previously stated that she avoided looking at herself in the mirror, and justified this by saying that one of her qualities was that she had never been particularly ‘vain’; therefore she equated looking in the mirror with ‘vanity’. In her mind, this changed Priscilla’s avoidant behaviour into a ‘quality’.

Creating her body image in clay must have been a challenge for Priscilla, as the clay sculpture can be seen as a ‘mirror’, reflecting all that she tried to avoid seeing. However, exploring her body image through clay in a supportive therapeutic environment, with an empathic listener, perhaps gave Priscilla the ‘permission’ to face her body image issues for the first time. Also, being in a group in study one with other women who were also facing body image issues, may have given Priscilla, Nancy, and Cynthia feelings of ‘solidarity’ and ‘community,’ something which can reduce feelings of alienation and encourage self-compassion.

This study has highlighted the impact mothers’ negative body image can have on their daughters. The reflections by Cynthia, Priscilla, and Nancy demonstrate the ways in which they were affected by their mother’s criticism, as well as their mother’s criticism of their own and other’s bodies.

7 Case Studies, Study Two

Clay Work as Meaningful Play

Priscilla, Cynthia, and Nancy: Clay Work as *Meaningful Play*

Within this chapter the case studies, drawn from Study Two of Dr Trisha Crocker's PhD research project, featuring the work of Priscilla, Cynthia, and Nancy, are presented and discussed in relation to the theme of clay work as *meaningful play*. Meaningful play within research and therapy utilises specific materials or games in order to elicit specific information or meaning from a situation or issue. The specific use of clay to explore body image is an example of how the choice of art materials within meaningful play can be chosen with a view to eliciting a more embodied response from the participants. For the purposes of this study, we define meaningful play as a playful activity which includes elements specifically chosen to elicit new learning and build meaning; it is therefore suitable for both research and therapy.

Priscilla

At many points during the sessions, the participants made explicit references to the way that they were manipulating the clay. In this instance Priscilla seemed to disconnect from her feelings as she cut away and added clay to different areas of her sculpture (see Figures 39 on p.105 & 41 on p.118), putting a lot of energy and thought into her work as she deliberated on the best tactics to use. Pausing constantly and devising an approach to construct her body image sculpture, Priscilla spoke of perhaps using 'an engineering' tactic.

> "So, what do [pause] – so, I could do that, and then I could say, well, I don't know [pause]. I don't know . . . go for the engineering approach? [pause]. I'll leave the back bit. It doesn't want to go out [pause]. I've often thought about this. I suspect the two halves then won't meet, which could actually be a bit of a problem."
>
> *Priscilla*

Art Therapist/Researcher Reflective Diary

As an empathic witness I was able to feel and reflect on Priscilla's changing attitude towards her body image sculpture, and I wondered if, with her first degree in engineering, Priscilla was either consciously or unconsciously selecting a discipline that she was familiar with which might create less emotional connection with her body image sculpture.

Offering the participants an opportunity to change their body image sculptures into something that more closely represented their body image was difficult for some. Here Priscilla seems attached to her old negative body image story, demonstrating her reluctance or fear of "destroying the bit that I do know".

> "Well, that doesn't really work, does it? No, well, I'm stuck because I can't really make it into something that I don't know without destroying the bit that I do know, and that's why I've never done anything about it."
>
> *Priscilla*

Saying "I can't really make it into something that I don't know without destroying the bit that I do know" suggested that Priscilla was beginning to recognise her resistance to change, and perhaps a feeling of comfort in "the bit that I do know". There was also the suggestion that Priscilla found it difficult to reconcile the fact that she could change her image, without destroying the parts she had grown to live with and to know. If she changed her sculpture, she would be changing her long-held self-perception. This may be an indicator as to why Priscilla had been unable to make changes to her body image in reality.

Playing with the clay by cutting it away and sticking it back on, Priscilla began to contemplate on what the outcome would be:

> "And since I don't want to leave today without all my bits, because that would perhaps start a precedent, which I wouldn't really quite like [pause]. What were those bits? That's not going to fit . . ."
>
> *Priscilla*

Attempting to change her image to something more realistic, and the tension this created between Priscilla's previous body image continued, but she seemed to want to work with the clay and to think through what it was that she could 'cut off' and leave behind. Still adding and taking away small pieces of clay from her work, Priscilla finally completed her image (see Figure 43).

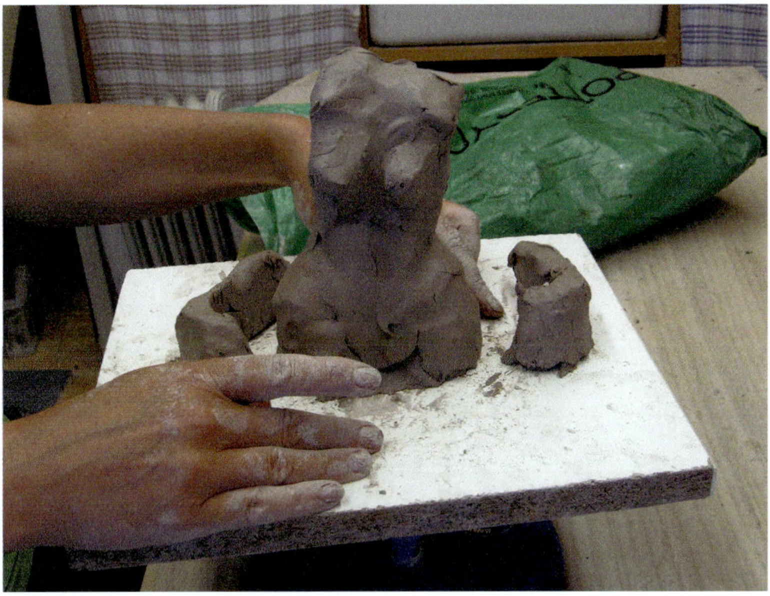

Figure 43 Sculpture No. 2 by *Priscilla.*
"There You Go . . . I've Lost an Inch!"

> "Yeah, and I suppose it's true. It's all true, but it's not to scale. Right, there you go. Possibly a better representation [pause]. Stick it here. Hey-ho, stick it here. Stick it – it's actually, you know alright, I can use half of that clay [pause]. It's an instant weight-loss program, fantastic [pause]. Now, I don't know where to stop [pause]. That bit sticks out a lot more. That sticks out a bit there [pause]. Bit of a tummy going on [pause]. That'll do. There you go. I've lost an inch. Excellent."
>
> *Priscilla*

Whilst sticking clay on to her sculpture and then scraping it off again, Priscilla stuck a smaller amount back on and exclaimed, "I can use half of that clay." There is a suggestion that using the clay to visualise her true image had led to a 'better representation'. As she said a "bit of a tummy going on" and then pausing to state "that'll do" alluded to a change of perception.

Nancy

When reviewing her clay body image sculptures, Nancy began to compare their shapes (see Figure 44 on p.126). The differences in colour and size were largely due to being at different stages of drying out and firing. The image on the right was Nancy's first sculpture, and already fired having been made in Study One. The sculpture in the middle was the first made in Study Two and drying

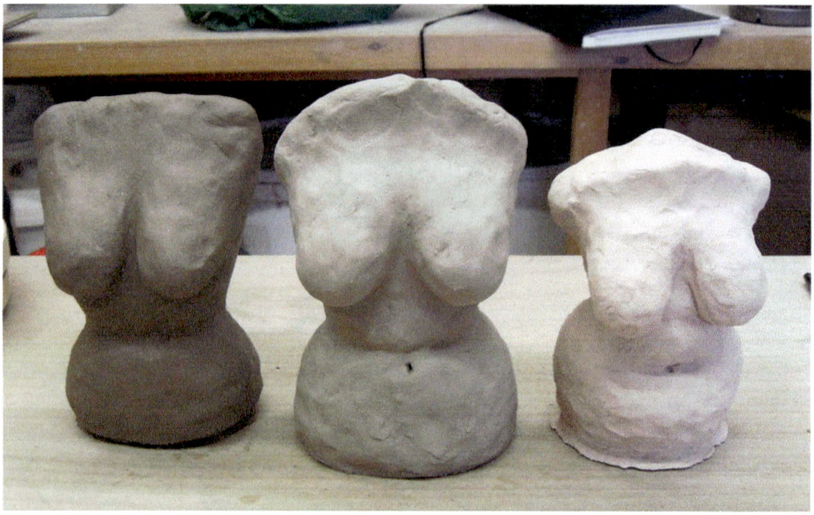

Figure 44 Sculptures Nos. 1, 2 & 3 by *Nancy.*
"The Three Nancys."

out ready for firing, and the darker one on the left was the second from Study Two and still visibly wet.

> "That one's very similar, although my tummy has popped out a little bit at the bottom [laughter], which I need to put on this one [laughs]. But yeah, my tummy goes in and out as it needs to."
>
> *Nancy*

While Nancy exclaimed that her "tummy has popped out a little bit at the bottom," she was actively lifting and tucking the clay, therefore using the clay as a means of intervention.

Art Therapist/Researcher Reflective Diary

Nancy's words about her tummy suggested that she was accepting her tummy needed to be realistic and to 'go in and out'.

As Nancy compared her clay sculptures, she attempted to refer to them as acceptable representations of herself but struggled to find the means and appeared unable to accept either of her clay body images as representing her body as she perceived it:

> "Because that's – that one is all bunched up and yeah, it's just not very nice at all, whereas when I saw it, when I was doing it here, I was actually really pleased with it. And I thought, well, if that's my body, that's my body, and that's okay. So, I was all right with that. But then, when I came back, I didn't like it. And again, this morning, I'm looking at it, going, God, that's just not my body."
>
> *Nancy*

Art Therapist/Researcher Reflective Diary

I wondered if Nancy was looking for what she emotionally perceived as 'perfection' and that her cognitive-focused approach was in conflict with her emotions . . .

> ". . . that's interesting, because actually, my body hasn't changed. My body doesn't really change. I'm going to put nipples on today. I've made a conscious decision [laughter]. My body hasn't – really, the integral shape of my body hasn't changed over the years. It's probably slightly different from my early 20s, but I didn't really appreciate what I had back then. And probably, actually, I'm bigger and lumpier than I was back then, and actually, I prefer my body – well, I like my body better than I did when in my 20s."
>
> *Nancy*

This may indicate that Nancy was finding more acceptance for her body as she aged, or that social pressure to conform to body image norms were less of an issue for her as an 'older' woman.

Nancy continued playing with the clay while reflecting:

> "I'm never happy with my boobs when I do them. I don't know what that's about?"
>
> *Nancy*

In session one Nancy said she 'liked' her breasts. Here she questions why she could not make her 'boobs' appear as she would like, and why they were still without nipples:

> "Yeah, and I put them [the nipples] on and I didn't like it. I think that's more aesthetics than anything else. I like the smooth shape. It's more

> like – I don't think – I'm not going to put a bum crack on it this time. I like the element of smoothness."
>
> *Nancy*

The word 'smooth' was used often by participants to describe their experience of touching and playing with the clay. For Nancy and Cynthia, the term could be a metaphor for each woman's desire to 'smooth out their lives'.

Nancy continued to cut at her clay body image saying:

> "What I'm just about to do is to chuck that bit up there [laughter]. Oh, dear. Take it off my [pause] . . . and put it on my boobs."
>
> *Nancy*

Early on in the session, 'chucking' the clay on and off the image, Nancy became focused on re-arranging herself. Laughing as she moved 'bits' around, she suggested that she could see the pointless aspects of worrying about such trivial differences she had previously perceived as important.

> "Oh, my goodness [pause]. I actually prefer the one in the middle, even though I'm saying that's a bit more [pause] – they are quite different, aren't they? They're the same, but different. I hate that one now [the first one]. Isn't that funny?"
>
> *Nancy*

Art Therapist/Researcher Reflective Diary

I wondered about Nancy publicly admitting that she 'hates' an image of her own body, perhaps the image she referred to appeared 'older' than the others, as the breasts appear more stretched than the other two. . . . This did serve to highlight that Nancy seemed to have a 'love/hate' relationship with her body image/sculpture.

Nancy spoke about her second sculpture, while comparing again her three sculptures (see Figure 40 on p.113). She decided the second one was the one that she liked best. Earlier, she had thought the first one was "gorgeous" and then remarked "I hate that now". Nancy's work with the clay had led to reflection and a suggestion that perhaps she could be happy with a more realistic body image, which spoke more about acceptance. Finally, she chose her second sculpture as the one she felt most represented her own body image.

> "Yeah, and it's not, not now I'm seeing it again [pause]. Not that that matters, because it's just, like, an image, but it's just [pause] – yeah, it's quite odd. But I still prefer that one. I think that one's much more me."
>
> *Nancy*

Art Therapist/Researcher Reflective Diary

I wondered if Nancy's attempt to enlarge the breasts on her third image, and then her realisation 'that isn't right', suggested the beginning of a more realistic awareness of her own body image.

Nancy was beginning to accept the lumps and bumps on her second image as being a more realistic representation of her body image, as she announced: "I think that one's much more me."

After reminding Nancy that we had discussed the lack of nipples on her image in the previous session, she talked about the intimacy of nipples:

> "They're strange little things and they're mine [laughter]. So, yeah, I'm not sure. I couldn't – and that was something I went away with last session, was just thinking, why didn't I put nipples on my boobs? And then I thought, well, I don't know. But then, I look at people's boobs up there [on the pottery shelf], and a lot of people haven't."
>
> *Nancy.*

Nancy also focused on what her nipples meant to her:

> "Yeah, I think I – when last – when we were talking about it last time, nipples, to me, are really intimate. And therefore, I'm not, kind of – I don't really know whether I want to put nipples on [laughs] . . ."
>
> *Nancy*

Nancy seemed reluctant to 'sexualise' her body image, and was perhaps also influenced by body image sculptures created by other participants that were on the drying rack in the studio, noticing that some of these had also been created without nipples, thereby finding confirmation and solidarity.

Art Therapist/Researcher Reflective Diary

I wondered if Nancy found something embarrassing or too intimate about creating and adding (and therefore displaying) her nipples, although she seemed able to speak about them without discomfort.

When comparing her new body image sculpture to the previous two she had made (see Figure 40 on p.113), Nancy was able to refer back to her previous work and reflect on any changes made. The image Nancy made in the second study she described as 'much bigger' than the first (at centre of Figure 44 on p.126), saying the first was 'absolutely gorgeous'.

When contemplating her final image, Nancy declared that she would put nipples on this; however, in the end, she didn't. As Nancy continued to reflect, she talked about the sameness and differences of her pieces.

Art Therapist/Researcher Reflective Diary

I wondered if this suggested contradiction and confusion because Nancy also said, "It's probably slightly different from my early 20s, but I didn't really appreciate what I had back then." I reflected that perhaps she was beginning to recognise herself in her sculpture and use it as a 'clay mirror'.

> "But it's smooth, and I like the smooth rather than [pause] – and it does seem that, when I concentrate on one element, like, everything else falls apart. It's like I can't do all the [laughs] things at once. It's like, I've been really focusing on, you know, sort of, exfoliating my skin and making it all nice and lovely. But then, my eating is rubbish [laughter] and it's like, when my eating was great, my skin felt awful because I wasn't moisturising – well, I was, I moisturise every day, but I wasn't kind of, doing this. Maybe, yeah, maybe I have a problem with doing two things at once [laughter]."
>
> *Nancy*

For Nancy, reflections on the state of her skin became an important subject:

> "And I think that maybe reflects that I've been really concentrating on my skin, trying to get all the rough bumps off my skin. So, maybe this is a little bit idealistic, because this is how I want my skin to be, all lovely and smooth and I'm only just working towards that at the moment, because my skin is really bad."
>
> *Nancy*

There was an implication that Nancy was beginning to notice that her perceptions were 'idealistic', rather than realistic, and may have helped her to let go of restrictive beliefs around needing to be 'perfect'.

> "Yeah, I think that is quite idealistic, actually. There's a little bit of reality, but I think that there is . . . that it's quite idealistic. But I like the idea of it being lovely and smooth."
>
> *Nancy*

As Nancy worked on her clay sculpture, she went through the process of building up and adding to the clay on her sculpture's breasts, knowing that she could change her impression of them with the clay, thinking about her shape with and without a bra:

> "And my boobs are probably a little bit more lifted. That's probably how they look when they're in the bra [laughs], rather than what they actually are. They're not as pointy as that outwards. They go down. So, I think there is a little bit of how I might look if I'm wearing my bra [pause]."
>
> *Nancy*

For Nancy there seemed to be a tension between being realistic and being idealistic when creating her body image sculpture.

Art Therapist/Researcher Reflective Diary

I wondered if the thoughts Nancy expressed were relevant to her previous thinking and processing her body image in a cognitive-focused way.

Nancy seemed to be attempting to create a 'realistic' reflection of her body image in her sculpture, but was unable to change it because for her this meant developing something 'idealistic'. For Nancy to reject creating a more 'idealistic' body image, in favour of 'reality', could be seen as a step towards acceptance, as it meant that Nancy was no longer trying to 'hide' or 'cover' it, or focus on a need for 'perfection'.

Although Nancy found aspects of her image idealistic, she liked it being 'lovely and smooth'. She then compared the three images (see Figure 44 on p.126), describing them either as ideal or more realistic, and viewed them all as very different even though they seemed quite similar:

> "I think that's more of an ideal, and I think that's more realistic. That's just maybe – because that – the top bit is a lot taller there. I don't know. Now I'm seeing that, that doesn't look like me at all, so I don't know what's happened there."
>
> *Nancy*

Art Therapist/Researcher Reflective Diary

I reflected that perhaps Nancy was unable to be happy with the body image she had created because it was a mirror for her own body image, something she did not like or accept, and therefore the sculpture was never going to be 'good enough'.

As Nancy studied her three sculptures, she came to the conclusion that they were all very similar but different, and she was most comfortable with the one which she felt resembled her most, even though it was the one that was not smooth, nor perfect in her eyes.

> "Yeah, that's a lot more petite there and . . . I don't know . . . I've always got this temptation to put this massive lump here, and my body isn't like that. That's more realistic, but that's still lumpy and bumpy."
>
> *Nancy*

This suggested that Nancy was beginning to accept her body image, discovering that she was not as big as she had perceived herself to be, but also not as 'smooth' as she would have liked.

Cynthia

Cynthia began the session by holding the lump of clay, turning it over in her hands and smoothing it, talking as she did so:

> "Because the thing I'm thinking and the thing I'm wanting to make at the moment, that is a completely blank, sort of . . . [pause] – a very serene, blank . . ."
>
> *Cynthia*

Art Therapist/Researcher Reflective Diary

Cynthia used the words 'blank' and 'serene' when talking about her sculptures. I wondered if this suggested that Cynthia was aiming to perhaps be relaxed and enjoy the experience of clay work without having to think too much. Perhaps she was aspiring to make a finished image that made her feel calm and without complications.

> "Then, it'll be something different. But as it changes, I suppose it reminds me of different things. And I'm thinking now of the Isles of Scilly. Do you know the Isles of Scilly?"
>
> *Cynthia*

Art Therapist/Researcher Reflective Diary

I was reflecting on the sensory nature of clay as I watched Cynthia working, which suggested to me that it was the sensation of the clay that was helping her to reflect.

Cynthia picked the clay up again after having put it down and talking some more, she began to make a block, and then to change it. She was turning the clay in her hands and the smoothness of the wet clay claimed her attention:

> "Yeah [pause], and I want to keep this smooth."
>
> *Cynthia*

As Cynthia smoothed and caressed the clay on her sculpture, she continued to speak about what the making of it meant to her:

> ". . . because there is that part, there's – there is that aspect. I've got a love of simplicity and peace and calm, and I think that's really – that's what this is about. And maybe this is my – this is an exterior . . . It's another façade, but it's also part of my holding myself together."
>
> *Cynthia*

Cynthia wanted to keep her image smooth on the outside. The cuts remained inside and at the top and there were holes to let light in (see Figures 33 & 34 on p.92).

Art Therapist/Researcher Reflective Diary

I reflected that Cynthia was working with her feelings, allowing the light to come in. By admitting that 'it's another façade' - she perhaps was stating that it is not an easy process to make change.

The wet and malleable clay allowed both Priscilla and Nancy to 'play' with the clay and channel their thoughts to 'reconstruct' their body image. They were then able to realise that their reconstructions were not so very different from how they desired to look.

This may have been the first time that Nancy felt safe enough to 'uncover' and talk about her body image issues, talking a great deal about her appearance while working with the clay. This suggests that working with clay in a meaningful way was a means of liberation for Nancy, allowing her the freedom to admit how she truly felt about her body image for the first time.

Section 3

Protocol, Evaluation Methods, and Conclusions – *Opening the Kiln*

8 Intervention Protocol

Aims of the Research Study

The main aim of the research study (Crocker 2017) was to ascertain the usefulness of clay work and the creation of a body image sculpture, as an art therapy tool for small groups of women or individuals to explore their body image issues.

Although hypothesis is not something that is usually part of an IPA qualitative study, there was a general belief that creating their body image sculpture, using the sensory and tactile material of clay, would be beneficial and could affect change for the participants. Giving participants the opportunity to view and discuss their body image sculptures within the group was also seen as a key part of this process.

The initial aim of Study One was to use it as a pilot study evaluating the ways in which clay might be used as a tool to explore body image in art therapy, including the advantages and disadvantages, and to collaboratively develop the protocol for this with participants through Action Research. It was also used to establish distinct questions for study two and to explore whether PAR or IPA was the best approach/method to use for the analysis.

Crank clay was used for all the sessions in each study, as it was considered the most suitable clay for body image sculptures, the unique plasticity of the clay making it particularly useful for slabbing and hand building techniques. The sculptures were photographed when wet, from each side, and then, once dried, they were fired with a 'bisque firing' of 1020c after which they were photographed again. Shrinkage of 5½% approximately is usual when clay dries, and then it is *bisque fired*, but as the participants mainly saw their sculptures in their original 'wet' form, shrinkage was not thought to be a significant issue.

For therapists who do not have access to a kiln, we would still recommend using crank clay for participants to use when sculpting their body image, even if the final pieces cannot be fired. Photographs can be taken of the objects to retain for further discussion and the sculptures then placed in special sealed bins to be recycled. We do not recommend the use of 'air drying clays' as this has a fibrous texture instead of the smooth silky texture. Similarly, the use of

Play-Doh® or Plasticine® are not considered as useful as real clay, as the sensory nature of playing with the clay is seen as important. However, further research is needed to see if the use of other materials is as effective as real clay.

The aims of Study One and Study Two were broadly the same, as the protocol from study one did not require significant change from one to the other. However, the wording was changed when introducing the study to participants, taking care to ask participants to create a sculpture in clay that reflected how they saw their own 'body image', rather than being a request to create a sculpture reflecting their own 'image'.

The aim of Study Two was to use the protocol developed through Study One for Study Two and develop a clear picture of how clay work can be an art therapy tool to help women explore their body image.

Venue for the Studies

The clay work sessions took place in 'The Pottery', a purpose-built Norwegian cabin situated at the far end of the researcher's garden. The Pottery contained

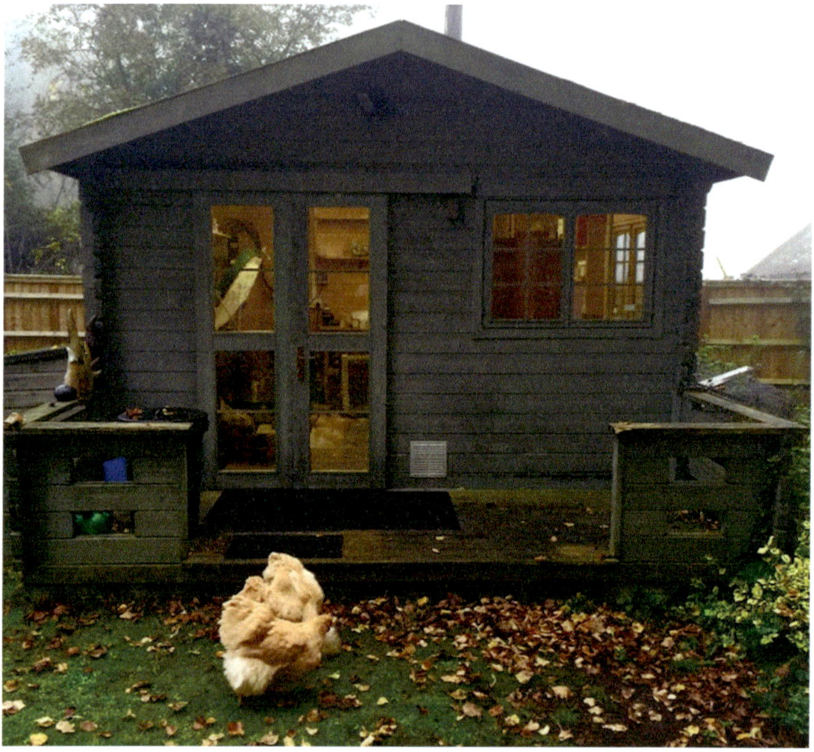

Figure 45 "The Pottery."

a sink, storage shelves for finished work, clay working tools, a large 4ft oval kiln, a rectangular table which seated four people comfortably – set in the centre of the room, and a side table under the windows seating two further people comfortably – and three if necessary.

The pottery was a warm and inviting space and offered a relaxing and welcoming workspace. The participants were offered refreshments prior to the session in a 'clean' area of the pottery, giving them the chance to get acquainted (although a couple of the participants in the first two sessions were known to each other). As cake was provided, this inevitably helped to open up the conversation about body image, calorie intake, etc.

It was important to create a confidential and boundaried space that felt 'safe' for the participants so that they would be able to explore their body image without feelings of fear or defensiveness. Participants were asked to turn off/silence their mobile phones and invited to wear aprons. The participants were not allocated a specific space; instead they selected their own spaces at the workbenches.

Ethical Approval and Considerations

The whole study was grounded in a rigorous ethical approach to ensure the safety of individual participants and their artworks. The main ethical issues to consider were confidentiality and dual-role conflict (Hart & Crawford-Wright, 1999; Martin et al. 2007). These have therefore been central considerations in the design of the project and the methods engaged, and the British Association of Art Therapists' (BAAT) ethical procedures were used as a guide to ensure participant and researcher safety throughout the study. Dual-role conflict (i.e. being both a therapist and researcher) was mitigated through ongoing supervision and reflexivity.

Ethical approval for the study was gained from the University of Derby Research Ethics Committee. Informed consent forms were signed by each participant, and contained information explaining how the clay images created by participants and recorded data from the sessions would be used and stored securely, as well as how information provided would be disseminated, e.g. within the PhD thesis, educational publications, and exhibitions. The names of the women were changed in all of the data collected throughout the study to ensure anonymity and confidentiality. The participants were also given or chose personalised identification numbers to inscribe into their images. This provided an anonymous way of identifying participants' work. The data collected from the two research studies was stored securely on a private computer.

As the majority of participants would be attending one-off sessions, the information provided to participants prior to the session informed them that if they had any questions, concerns, or reflections that they wanted to express in private with the facilitator at the end of the sessions, then she would be available for this. This was to ensure the safety of participants and ensure that each participant left feeling heard and understood, and not overwhelmed by the content of the sessions.

It is important when carrying out any art therapy work to attend regular supervision sessions with a trained therapist, and, particularly when conducting research, to develop a *reflexive* approach (Etherington 2004a; 2004b; 2004c) – in order to create transparency and to acknowledge one's own subjective 'internal and external responses', and 'cultural or theoretical constructs' (Etherington 2004b, p.46).

Clay Safety

The safety of participants was of utmost priority during sessions involving clay work. Participants were advised at the beginning of the clay making session that: food and drink was only to be consumed in the 'clean' area, not at the workbenches. Aprons and gloves were offered to those who required them. Handwashing facilities were available. Masks were not available for participants as they were only using wet clay, however they would have been used if dry or fired clay had been rubbed down with glass paper, as this can create a toxic dust.

Transcribing Recordings

The voice recordings from each session were sent to a professional transcriber (who guaranteed confidentiality) and transcribed them verbatim. To ensure additional confidentiality participants were referred to as Participant 1, 2, 3 . . . etc. on the recordings, and any identity revealing content was removed from the recordings before transcription. The voice recordings were then drawn upon when conducting the analysis to corroborate interpretations, 'essences', and themes that emerged from the visual data.

Photography

Photographs of the clay body image sculptures were taken as a back-up before the sculptures were fired in case of any breakages in the kiln, and photographed again at a higher resolution once the pieces were fired. These photographs were then used to aid discussion and analysis where the original three-dimensional forms were not present, and in order to enable analysis while working away from them.

Participant Recruitment

Careful purposive selection was used to help erect and maintain boundaries around the study. Women aged between 25 and 54 years, without a known diagnosis of eating disorders or body image issues or who had not previously expressed body image issues, were selected.

The participants were recruited from a range of local educational establishments, as well as colleagues and acquaintances of Trisha Crocker, most of whom were known to her only in passing. In the first instance an email was sent to potential participants, inviting them to take part in the study, and advising them that this would include making an image of themselves in clay and engaging in a recorded discussion about the process. 16 women from a wide range of backgrounds registered their interest in attending. Those that were able to attend on the dates offered took part in the sessions.

Criteria for Inclusion to the Study

Women over the age of 25 who had not previously identified as having an eating disorder or body image issues. Women of any ethnicity were included.

Criteria for Exclusion to the Study

As this study focused entirely on women's experience of body image, men were excluded from the study. Women under the age of 25 were also excluded as the focus was on women considered 'mature' in age. Women who identified themselves as currently or previously experiencing an eating disorder or body image issues for which they had sought therapy or medical intervention were also excluded.

Study One: The Pilot Study

Study One acted as a pilot study, used to inform the protocol and methods of analysis for Study Two. The main changes between Study One and Study Two were the importance of using consistent language, e.g. inviting participants to create their own 'body image', rather than 'image' and the decision to use IPA as a research methodology.

A humanistic, person-centred approach (Rogers 2003 [1951]) to art therapy was followed during the sessions, to enable the development of empathic and authentic therapeutic relationships. This approach requires the forming of a therapeutic alliance based on: empathic understanding, unconditional positive regard, psychological contact, therapist authenticity, and relational depth based on trust (ibid.). This approach ensured that the participants felt heard and free from judgment.

When the participants arrived, they were advised about the requirement for them all to agree to keep the contents of the session confidential. They were also advised about therapist/researcher's limits on confidentiality, saying that any issues raised that could result in themselves or someone they know being harmed, would be reported to the correct authorities. A brief description of the study and their role within it was given, along with their right to withdraw from the study at any time. Participants were then given the opportunity to ask any questions and then invited to complete an informed consent form.

Study One consisted of four sessions involving 16 women aged between 25 and 57 years, who each attended one of the four sessions. The group size fluctuated due to the personal commitments of the participants. As Study One served as a pilot study for Study Two, we have discussed Study One on its own in order to provide a clear picture of the way the protocol was developed for Study Two.

Study One, Session One: Participants

Helena, was a 42-year-old woman who identified as British/Asian. Helena had a post-graduate degree in fine art. Helena was married, and at the time of the sessions her daughter was soon to be a teenager. Helena was brought up in the UK by her English grandmother, her parents were divorced and living in Asia. Helena spoke openly to the group about having experienced two late miscarriages.

Sarah was a 48-year-old white British woman, divorced, and a mother of two primary school- age children. Sarah was also a Doctor.

Victoria was a 48-year-old, white British woman, divorced, and a mother of two adult sons. Victoria had recently been trained and employed within a county borough as a family/child worker.

Linda was a 56-year-old, white British woman, married, and mother to an 18-year- old daughter. Linda was a trained massage therapist.

Veronica was a 52-year-old white British woman, divorced and mother to a girl and a boy of primary and secondary age. Veronica held a diploma in art, had attended ballet classes for many years, and was involved in a local amateur dramatic group.

Nancy was a single 34-year-old white British woman, working for a borough council as a trained child/family worker.

Study One, Session Two: Participants

Jenny was a 44-year-old white British woman, married and a mother to two adopted children of primary age. Jenny had held a high-powered job when she had met her husband. Together they owned a large house in the country. Jenny was also a carer for her parents, who were unwell and lived a long distance away.

Edina was a 41-year-old white British woman, married and mother to two sons. Edina was working as a florist and married to an artist.

Willow was a 25-year-old white British woman (the youngest participant to attend the study). Willow's mother had gone through many operations to change the shape of her body.

Priscilla was a 51-year-old white British woman, married and mother to three teenage girls.

Priscilla's family did not own a television for the majority of the children's school years so that their childhood would not be exposed to outside influences the parents could not control. They aimed as parents to give the children a wide variety of skills and interests both inside and outside of the home. Priscilla had been an engineer before having her children.

Jane was a 57-year-old white British woman, married and mother to one son, who was at college. Jane worked as a teacher of profoundly handicapped children.

Study One, Session Three: Participants

Eleanor was a 47-year-old white Canadian woman, married, and mother to a boy and girl of primary school age. Eleanor was employed as a senior manager for a large international company and held an MA and MBA. Eleanor's husband, who was 20 years her senior, was a house-husband. Eleanor and her husband, who were originally from Canada, were planning to return there to live.

Paula was a 39-year-old white British woman, single, with no children, working as a primary school teacher and hypnotherapist.

Participants in Study One Attending Both Sessions, Three and Four

Justine was a 47-year-old white British, married, mother of two boys of primary age, who was working as an editor.

Sunny was a 41-year-old British/Asian woman, born in India, married to an English man and mother to three primary school age children (primary age). Sunny was an engineer before she left to become a full-time mother.

Cynthia was a 52-year-old white British woman, a trained nurse and a mother to two adult children. Cynthia had been separated from her husband for a number of years, but due to necessity they were still living in the same house.

Session Protocol Study One

Study One consisted of six group sessions in total, each with four–six participants. Study Two consisted of three individual sessions. The sessions were three hours long in total, with the first hour dedicated to clay work and the second hour to discussion, followed by a written questionnaire to be completed by participants.

On arrival participants were offered tea, coffee, and cake within the 'clean area' of the pottery studio, which consisted of a table and chairs. Participants were also given a form to complete asking for their: age, ethnicity, highest level of education, profession, country of birth married/partner, single, other sexual preference, if they had children, and any other information that they would like to share relevant to the study. These questions were chosen as they were considered relevant to a study on body image.

The Clay Work

No instructions were given to the participants regarding techniques on how to create their image with clay. Instead the participants were encouraged to 'play' and build their sculptures instinctively. Most of the participants said they had not used clay since they were at school.

The participants began the clay sculpture-making process by cutting pieces of clay from a large bag of crank clay which was on each table. Participants were therefore able to select a lump of clay to make their sculpture and take more out of the bag if needed. Wooden clay working tools were also available for the participants to use, e.g. cutting, scraping, smoothing, and marking tools.

Participants also had access to a large selection of clay working tools, water, and sponges for smoothing. The body image sculpture-building session lasted for one hour, with time reminders being given at 20-, 10-, and 5-minute intervals towards the end of the hour, to ensure that participants had time to complete their sculptures. Once the participants had completed their sculpture, they then washed their hands and went to the clean area to make themselves a cup of tea or coffee and have a piece of cake if they chose to.

This was followed by a one-hour focus group discussion about the process of making the clay sculptures, the body images participants had created, and their meanings. The one-hour time allowance given to the discussion proved to be sufficient for reflection and contemplation. The participants used the time to express similar doubts and insecurities about their body images, and to reflect on this together. It was felt that restricting the time ensured that each participant had time for their own personal reflection, but did not allow anxiety to build up within the group, as there was insufficient time for this to be addressed in a one-off session. However, it was made clear to the group that anyone who wanted to talk privately with the art therapist after the session or at a later date would be given the opportunity to do so.

The focus group discussions were recorded and transcribed verbatim. As well as listening to the discussions during the clay work and focus group sessions, observations were also made and field notes taken by the therapist/researcher, regarding participants' body placements, emotion, and language used. The therapist/researcher also ensured that the discussion focussed on body image, and was brought back to topics deemed 'safer' when dialogue strayed to areas considered 'unsafe'. These included e.g. participants focusing on one particular group member's weight problems and giving advice about diets/lifestyle changes that were not necessarily appropriate.

End of Session Questionnaire

At the end of each session the participants were invited to complete a questionnaire about their experience of making their clay body image sculpture and the discussion.

Open-ended questions were predominately used in order to allow the participants space to direct the subject matter towards their own experience of the phenomenon and address issues that were important to them, allowing for the emergence of unanticipated themes and understandings (Smith, Flowers & Larkin 2009).

Questions from the End of Session Questionnaire:

1. What did you hear me ask of you before you began?
2. How did you begin the work? What were your thought processes?
3. How does the image represent you?
4. Did your feelings change over the session as you worked with the clay?
5. If yes, how and when did your feelings change?
6. What was it like to use the clay?
7. Do you think the experience would have been the same if you had drawn or painted your image on paper? Please explain.
8. Do you think the three-dimensional image was a factor in the thought process? Please explain.
9. Would you like to add any other thoughts about the process of using the clay?
10. Would you say the process was intimidating, cathartic, thought provoking, or other? Please explain in as much detail as you can.
11. Did working on your own enhance the process after working in a group, or make no difference? Please explain.
12. Did discussing your work on a one to one with a trained art therapist make a difference to the experience?
13. If you had made the image on your own, in your own environment, do you feel you would have gained as much, more, or less, understanding of your feelings? Please explain.
14. Would you like to add anything else?
15. How could this experience have been made better?
16. If you have been asked to make a second sculpture of your 'ideal' self, please discuss and compare the two. Were they very different from each other?

These questions are from the individual sessions (as you can see from questions 11 and 12). In the group sessions the following questions were used instead of 11 and 12.

- Did working in a group enhance the process or make a difference? Please explain.
- Did discussing your work within the group make a difference to the experience?

The participants wrote their replies prior to leaving the session; however, they were also invited to write an email about their experience and any further thoughts they had about the process, and send them to the therapist/

researcher. This gave the participants time for further reflection on the process and their experience. These further thoughts have also been included in the analysis.

Study Two

Participants for Study Two consisted of three women aged between 34 and 54 years, who had all also taken part in Study One, they were: Nancy, Priscilla, and Cynthia. Each attended individual clay work sessions in Study Two. Of the three women selected for Study Two, one was married, one divorced, and one was single, offering a diverse selection of relationship experience. The participants chosen for Study Two were selected because of their keen interest in contributing to the next stage of the research, their ability to verbalise clearly their thought processes while working with clay, and their availability to attend Study Two. Unfortunately, neither of the two British women from Study One with an Asian heritage were able to attend Study Two.

The sessions in Study Two were all one-off individual sessions that lasted for two and a half to three hours.

The protocol developed in Study One (the pilot study), was used for Study Two; however, the wording for the initial instructions was changed from 'make an image of yourself in clay' to 'make a body image sculpture of yourself in clay'. There was also a difference in that the three women selected for Study Two had already attended a group session in Study One; they were therefore already familiar with the surroundings and protocol, and had begun the process of thinking about their body image and how it could be represented in clay.

The pilot study also served to review the effectiveness of the protocol and confirm that it worked as a vehicle for women who were interested in exploring their body image through clay. Very little therefore needed to be changed for Study Two; however, a question was added to the post-session questionnaire asking about participants' experience of working one to one, after working in a group:

> "Did working on your own enhance the process after working in a group, or make no difference? Please explain."

The participants were given one hour to complete their body image sculptures, and were given time warnings of the ending of the hour at 20-, 10-, and 5-minute intervals. Study Two differed from Study One in that the three women were invited to modify their final sculptures if they wished, to make them more a reflection of reality. Most had already finished by the end of the session and tidied up, washed their hands, and were enjoying a cup of tea/coffee and cake. (Some said 'I shouldn't' and then helped themselves to more cake!).

Finally, the participants were then invited to complete a questionnaire about their experience of creating their clay body image sculptures, and the discussion groups. Some of the participants also sent emails/letters describing further thoughts on their experience, once they had reflected upon it.

Action Research

Action Research (AR) (Reason & Bradbury 2008; Chevalier & Buckles 2013) was chosen as the design method for study one (pilot study). AR can be described as a 'democratic and participative orientation to knowledge creation. It brings together action and reflection, theory and practice, in the pursuit of practical solutions to issues of pressing concern' (Bradbury 2008, p.1). AR is a qualitative research method where collaboration is encouraged so that research is undertaken *with* participants rather than *on* participants (Bradbury 2008, p.1). Action, followed by reflection and reflexivity, are also important aspects of action research (ibid.), therefore in this research the results of Study One were used to inform the protocol for Study Two. The iterative design of Study One meant that following the sessions, reflections and small changes were made, e.g. adopting an Interpretative Phenomenological Analysis methodology for the analysis of data from Study Two.

Study One used some aspects of Participatory Action Research (PAR) in that it encouraged participants to discuss the processes involved in the study, through the focus group discussions, in order to inform Study Two. Changes implemented included the suggestion from participants to make the opening instructions clearer for participants.

During the clay work sessions participants related to each other as women and companions in order to search for self-knowledge and understanding – through reflecting on their body image and relating stories of self-identity relating to their body image. Sally Skaife (2000) reiterates peer support processes in art therapy groups: 'In the group, members relate to each other as companions in the pursuit of art, and/or in the stories that have brought them to therapy' (p.121). Marian Liebmann (1997) also cites peer support as important for womens' empowerment within art therapy groups.

Field Notes

Reflections on each of the participants' attitudes and body language were noted in the field notes immediately after the session, as were important words, themes, or aspects of the session. Field notes were written during and after sessions. Data was then further reflected upon and noted in the reflective diary.

Reflective Diary

This diary was a place for reflective and reflexive writing and note-taking, enabling the identification of themes, connections, and meanings in the clay work sessions and discussion. Intuitive and resonant thoughts about the creative process were recorded, as were reflections on the participants' experience of the project. A reflexive and reflective approach should not be confused with removing *subjectivity*, as this is something that cannot and should not be erased from the creative process, rather 'subjectivity should be engaged with as a central aspect of ethnographic knowledge, interpretation and representation' (Pink 2007, p.23). Willig (2010, p.10) describes reflexivity as having two dimensions, the personal and the epistemological. Personal reflexivity is about reflecting on the ways in which our own values, experiences, wider aims, identities, and interests have shaped the research, and epistemological reflexivity depends upon our engaging with questions about how the research has been constructed (ibid.).

Observation and field note-taking was one of the key methods used to monitor the ways in which the clay and image making was approached by the participants. Changes and modifications that the participants made during the clay work session were also recorded, as well as their body language and any physical expressions made as they talked. Information from the reflective diary was used within the analysis; however, this was 'bracketed' within the 'Art Therapist/Researcher Reflective Diary' statements.

The diary was divided into four sections (Hughes 2006; Baxter et al. 2001):

1. Observational notes describing the clay making sessions and observations of what took place without interpretation.
2. Methodological notes reflecting on the clay work sessions,
3. Theoretical notes to begin making meaning of the data.
4. Analytical notes bringing together the observations, methodologies, and theory, while linking these to any published research in the field.

Whilst the participants were creating their clay sculptures, reflections and field notes were made in the diary. Witnessing the women as they created their body image sculptures, and listening to the way in which words were articulated as they examined and discussed their completed clay pieces, were also key processes that were added to the reflective diary to inform the analysis. The diary also served as a space to record personal reflective and reflexive thoughts on the clay work process and the discussions that took place on their completion. It was also a place to consider the underlying phenomena of personal interpretations, and defend against possible researcher bias.

Developing a New Protocol for Art Therapy Practice and Future Studies in this Field

Through revisiting the data, we have developed a new protocol, that utilises important learning from both Study One and Study Two. The aim is for clients to attend an initial series of *meaningful play* group art therapy sessions, with women of similar ages and life experiences, to create clay sculptures that reflect their body images. A group of between four and six women would be recommended.

The objectives of the intervention were for women to use the clay sculptures as visual and metaphoric body image representations, that enabled their stories of embodiment to be remembered, developed, and recognised, through the use of metaphor, symbolism, and realism, and a process of being authentically seen. This meant offering and receiving peer support from the other women in the group and developing feelings of self-compassion and healing for body-shame, through finding points of connection and solidarity in the body image stories of the other women.

- In the first session, invite each participant to create an *abstract*, non-figurative sculpture of their body image, as this will encourage the use of *metaphor and symbolism* to weave stories of body image, over and around and through the sculptures. Inviting participants to create an 'abstract' sculpture is non-threatening as it does not require figurative sculptural skills and may encourage the cathartic use of the clay. Historical body image issues, critical mothers and others, and perfectionism are all issues to look out for by the art therapist, whilst also acting as a companioning empathic witness and a safe-guarding presence within the group.
- After the clay work in each session schedule a one-hour discussion time, giving time for each woman within the group to share stories around their abstract body image sculpture. This enables the members of the group to make connections between their own sculpture and the other stories of body image shared by the group, encouraging feelings of solidarity.
- Give each participant a small sketchbook/journal to write or draw in at home, noting any experiences relevant to their body image they identify post session or during the week if sessions are weekly. This can then be brought into subsequent group discussions.
- Within the second session the participants should be invited to create a *figurative* representation of their body image. Some brief guidance on clay sculpting skills would be helpful before this session commences to ensure participants are not left feeling frustrated by a lack of skill.
- The women are then invited to discuss these figurative sculptures in the discussion time after the session, and to note whether their sculptures are an accurate representation.
- On the third session the women should be invited to create a final sculpture that incorporates the learning from the first two sessions and create a more accurate *revisioning* of their body image, to ensure that each feels *authentically seen* by the other group members.
- The final discussion will bring together the three sculptures made by each of the group members, with the opportunity to note the similarities and relationships between all the sculptures created, so as to develop a group story of body image, something that this project has shown helps develop feelings of self-compassion and solidarity between the women.

- It is important for the group members to be offered further one-to-one art therapy clay work sessions following the group sessions, as these may be needed to further develop new positive body image stories and feelings of self-compassion.

Through revisiting the data, we were able to re-evaluate the information from Study One and Study Two and develop a protocol that reflects the best practice from both studies. Our aim is to offer a protocol that will provide the best outcomes for art therapy practice; however, we recognise that people are individuals with differing needs, and therefore, as with other art therapy interventions, the protocol will need to be flexible and modified to suit the demographic of each individual client or groups of clients.

9 Methods of Analysis

This project employed clay work as a visual research method and intervention, and as Pink (2004) suggests, visual research can be used successfully in projects that

> [. . .] seek to represent the ways people experience certain dimensions of their everyday worlds and that create platforms on which people can represent their experiences, views, or culture. It facilitates the representation of embodied aspects of self [. . .], the use of metaphor and the empathetic communication of knowledge and experience that cannot be expressed using words alone.
>
> (p.10)

When selecting and adapting methods for analysis it was important to recognise that this equates to constructing a 'theoretical and ontological' filter through which to analyse the participants experience of body image (Mauthner & Doucet 1998, p.23). Whilst these choices affect the results achieved, the aim was for transparency, enabling other therapists and researchers to trace the procedures followed and reflexive decision-making processes (ibid.).

As the aim was to develop a simple and flexible study design within which to research, something as dynamic, complex, and personal as body image, Participatory Action Research (PAR) and Interpretative Phenomenological Analysis (IPA) were selected. This method of analysis was considered to be an effective way to answer the epistemological questions regarding what can be learned about women's body image issues through the use of clay work and the construction of a body image sculpture. It allowed for the explication of a qualitative search for 'meaning' and the condition and quality of the participants' experience, rather than identifying the cause and effects affecting a person's life (Willig 2010, p.8).

Participatory Action Research (PAR)

PAR was used for Study One, and acted as a pilot study enabling the methods to be developed and adjusted for Study Two. PAR is described as a method of research that involves a collaboration between researchers and participants, in an effort to understand together context-specific issues, and develop strategies to effect positive social change (Argyris 1999).

Participatory Action Research (PAR) is based on a process of *iteration*, meaning that within Study One cycles of intervention, reflection, and modification, were used (Avison et al. 1999; Hayes 2012). This meant that after each session the process, results, and feedback from participants (from field notes and participants questionnaire) were reflected upon and small adjustments were made to improve the following workshop.

Interpretative Phenomenological Analysis (IPA)

IPA was chosen as the approach/analysis method for Study Two, as this provided a structured approach to data collecting and collating, with a strong base for analysing transcripts of the sessions and interviews without bias. IPA is often used in qualitative social- and health-related inquiries, and is an important approach for examining how individual people make sense of significant life experiences (Smith, Flowers & Larkin 2009). IPA is underpinned by the phenomenological theories of Edmund Husserl (1977 [1929], 1970 [1954]) who believed that in order to identify the essential qualities of an experience one needed to 'go back to the things themselves'. This involves a process of phenomenological reduction, which includes 'bracketing out' the taken-for-granted world, in order to focus on a *conscious experience* of it (Giorgi 1992, p.114).

IPA thus focuses on the experience of participants, and engages with the way people reflect on the significance of that experience (Smith, Flowers, & Larkin 2009). IPA also features a *double hermeneutic* within its interpretative analysis, whereby the researcher attempts to interpret the participants accounts in order to understand their experience, whilst the participant is also attempting to understand their own experience (ibid.).

IPA blends both *phenomenological reduction* (Husserl 1977 [1929], 1970 [1954]) and *phenomenological hermeneutic interpretation* (Heidegger 1962 [1927]; Gadamer 1975), as a way to combine the *life* experience (i.e. a return to the things themselves through a reduction to essences) and the *world* (i.e. cultural and historic meanings and understandings) of lived experience. This recognises that experience or *life* does not happen in a vacuum, but is always situated within the *world.* IPA is also 'idiographic', in that it functions to discover in detail what the experience is like for a specific person, and what this specific person makes of their experience (Smith, Flowers & Larkin 2009, p.3). IPA research also employs the iterative method or 'hermeneutic circle', which includes a process of moving back and forth between different ways of thinking about the data (ibid. p.28).

As the aims of IPA studies include discovering in detail qualitative experiential data, they are generally conducted with relatively small numbers of participants – between 3 and 12 people is considered sufficient (Smith, Flowers & Larkin 2009). Smith, Flowers and Larkin (2009) suggest that between 4 and 10 participants for doctoral phenomenological research studies is generally sufficient. Due to the small number of participants IPA does not seek to generalise findings, but rather to offer insight into experience that can be used to inform practice, policy, and further research.

As IPA does not separate description from interpretation, the participant's life experiences are explored, alongside the researcher's own view of the world. Meaning that 'the interaction of researcher and participant are vital to the interpretation of the participant's experience' (Willig 2010, p.57), whilst also being mindful to avoid any projection of the therapist's/researcher's own personal ideas or issues. The aim was to bracket personal assumptions while witnessing the clay making and listening to what the women said so as to be free from projection and judgement as much as possible.

It was therefore vitally important that, during the discussions and interviews, participants were given the opportunity to explain the personal meaning they ascribed to their clay sculptures, and that extracts of the participants' verbatim narrative were used to support and corroborate any interpretation by the researcher (Smith, Flowers & Larkin 2009).

Because IPA involves close examination of the experiences and meaning-making activities of participants, a much more nuanced and detailed analysis of three individual participants was possible. As Henn, Weinstein & Foard (2006) say:

> Unlike positivism, the interpretive approach assumes that human behaviour is not determined by external factors and processes that researchers can measure, but instead is shaped by the meanings people have of the world. [. . .]The research therefore will tend to be small scale and intensive. It will also usually be flexible and relatively unstructured and based upon detailed descriptions (rather than statistics) of what is seen and heard.
>
> (p.15).

The aim of using IPA was to explore in detail how the study participants made sense of their world in a detailed and empathetic manner. Rather than attempting to definitively hypothesise, the aim was to explore the participant's experience of clay work and body image, with flexibility and an open mind. The use of IPA, involving the exploration of the personal experiences of the participants and the researcher along with the third account given by the visual clay content, therefore became the basis for the analysis.

Clay work and sculptures of the human form are both a social practice and an art form, and exist within a complex web of subject–object relations (Pointon 2013). By adding an interpretative aspect to phenomenological research, as in IPA, it is possible to situate the work within the life 'worlds' of the women creating their body image sculptures, and consider the influence cultural symbolism and metaphor have on this reflective and interpretative understanding (Lester 1999; Finlay 2011).

Multiple Case-Study Design

A case study can be defined as an 'empirical inquiry' which 'investigates a contemporary phenomenon within its real-life context; when the boundaries between phenomenon and context are not clearly evident; and in which multiple sources of evidence are used' (Yin 2009, p.23). A multiple case-study design was selected as it is a qualitative research method capable of incorporating both visual and verbal data (Yin 2012), and case studies can be particularly relevant for relational-centred approaches to phenomenological research (Finlay 2011).

In art therapy research the case study is a method of enquiry which is able to address the key aspects of clinical work, and the ability to focus on the 'individuality' of the client, embracing the 'richness, diversity, messiness and complexity' of the art making process and clients' lived experience. It doesn't require 'subjects' be turned into 'objects'; instead it encourages writing about clients in a way that is 'recognisably human' (Edwards 1999, p.6).

Within IPA a case study for each participant is developed individually and completed before continuing on to the next one (Smith, Flowers & Larkin 2009, pp.79–107). Within the case study the original transcripts relating to each participant are read more than once, exploring not only the content but the language used, etc. Emergent themes for this individual will begin to develop. Once all the case studies are completed a cross-case analysis can be carried out, where the themes from each case study can be compared and grouped by subject matter to form a cross-case analysis. These themes are then added to a master table of themes from all cases.

The focus of the cross-case analysis is therefore concerned with explicating the participants unique experiences, how these relate to the group as a whole, and the implications of this for wider contexts. Cross-case analysis also enables 'triangulation' between the cases and the drawing of convergent understandings (Yin 2012 p.13). Although it is only possible to make tentative generalisations from cross-case analysis (Smith, Flowers & Larkin, 2009) the relevance of one or more person's experience to others in a similar situation can be a key way that case studies gain validity (Hogan 1997).

IPA Thematic Analysis

As IPA uses idiography, which can be described as a focus on the particular rather than the universal (Smith, Harré & van Langenhove, 1995), in-depth case studies were created for each participant, including individual statements by the researcher/therapist and the identification of subordinate themes. While the main concern of IPA is to give a full account of each individual's experience, once all the case studies were completed, all the subordinate themes were examined, compared, and contrasted, demonstrating similarities and differences, in order to generate superordinate themes that appeared across the case studies (Pietkiewicz & Smith 2014, p.8).

The initial stage involved immersion in the data, through multiple close readings of the transcripts, as well as listening to the audio recordings to recall and recreate the atmosphere of the clay studio, and make further field notes and reflections in the reflective diary. Each reading/listening to the data provided new insights and notes of potential significance, e.g. topics discussed, language used, metaphors, symbolism, repetitions, emotion, context, etc. (Pietkiewicz & Smith 2014).

Analysing the participants' verbal and written transcripts was a complex and time-consuming activity; however, by totally immersing one's self in the data, the researcher/therapist is able to 'step into the participants' shoes as far as possible' (Pietkiewicz & Smith 2014, p.11), in order to document the participants' attempts to make sense of their body image sculptures.

Translating Data into Subordinate Themes

Data from the field notes and reflective diary was then used to identify emergent/subordinate themes and phrases, whilst also ensuring that these were grounded in the data from the participant's account, therefore representing the hermeneutic circle, where 'the part is interpreted in relation to the whole, and the whole is interpreted in relation to the part' (Pietkiewicz & Smith 2014, p.12). Sections from the verbatim transcripts, originating within the clay work sessions and interviews, were placed within tables for analysis, as outlined by Smith, Flowers and Larkin (2009).

Notes taken when observing a participant's body language as she worked with the clay, and listening to what was being revealed and how it was being articulated, as well as observing the finished product, provided a rich source of reflections on the meaning and significance of the phenomenon. Throughout the analysis process the clay body image sculptures belonging to each participant were visually referred to from each side.

Identifying Superordinate Themes: Finding relationships and Clustering Themes

In this part of the analysis subordinate/emergent themes identified from each case study were grouped together according to concept similarities and connections, and placed under a descriptive label. Some minor themes, with weak evidence base, were dropped at this stage. Once the superordinate themes were identified, the participant transcripts were revisited and relevant supporting extracts selected were listed alongside the themes, as corroborating evidence (Pietkiewicz & Smith 2014, p.130).

The Superordinate Themes	*Participants who Engaged with the Theme*
Altering Body Image Perception with the Use of Clay for Reflection	Priscilla, Nancy, and Cynthia
The Aging Body	Priscilla and Cynthia
Comparing Self to Others	Priscilla and Nancy
Emotional Affect, i.e. anger & sadness	Priscilla
Un-Met Expectations	Nancy and Cynthia
The Critical Mother	Priscilla, Nancy, and Cynthia
Body-Shame and Covering the Self	Nancy, Cynthia
Metaphor & Symbolism	Priscilla, Nancy, and Cynthia

These were then placed into a table with column headings for the coding, including: linguistic, conceptual, and descriptive.

Writing Up the IPA Study

IPA research studies require that a narrative account is written following the identification of themes. For this study this involved describing each individual theme identified, then including extracts from participants' verbal transcripts and images of the body image sculptures as supporting material, as well as analytic comments from the therapist/researcher. This enabled the production of an explanatory account explaining the important experiential learning and meanings discovered by the study (Pietkiewicz & Smith 2014, p.13). Using the participants' own words within the narrative description enables transparency and retains the voice of the participants, with the reader also able to use this to assess the congruity of the interpretations. The final description also includes elements of the interpretative analysis by the therapist/researcher and notes from the reflective diary; however, care is taken to ensure that the voices of the participant and that of the researcher/therapist are identified and separated. Finally, implications for further research and practice are identified.

As this book enabled further reflection and analysis, some of the themes originally identified within the research/therapist thesis (Crocker 2017) have been further developed and expanded upon, generating new insights. The combination of visual and verbal data ensured that corroboration was possible.

A Phenomenological Approach to Research and Analysis

Phenomenology can be simply described as a philosophical approach to gaining knowledge by examining the nature of consciousness through direct experience. Phenomenological research is 'discovery-orientated and offers a way of explicating the essential qualities and structures of art therapy phenomena' (Quail & Peavy 1994, pp.45).

Merleau-Ponty (quoted in van Manen 1990, p.13) described phenomenology as a 'poetizing project' which enables a 'primal telling', and a language that engages people's voices to 'sing the world' rather than 'abstractly speaking *of* it . . . so that *in* the words, or perhaps better, *in spite of* the words, we find "memories" that paradoxically we never thought or felt before' (van Manen 1990, p.13 [emphasis original]).

There are many threads to phenomenology; however, there are two main approaches which can broadly be described firstly as the Husserlian *transcendental* phenomenology (1970 [1945]; 1977 [1929]) which concentrates on the 'a return to the things themselves' or a pre-reflective, descriptive experience of the lived world, and secondly as Heidegger's (1962 [1927)] *hermeneutic* phenomenology which concentrates on a reflective interpretative consciousness, or 'seeking universal meaning' from lived experience (van Manen 1990, p.19). A hermeneutic phenomenology therefore acknowledges the meanings that sociocultural traditions give to the *lifeworld* (van Manen 1990, p.12). Importantly this meant that the sociocultural context within which the client developed her body image could also be explored and therefore part of the analysis.

Phenomenology employs a process of phenomenological reduction, 'which implies the bracketing of past knowledge about the phenomenon being experienced' (Giorgi 1992, p.114). Bracketing suggests a suspension of judgment, and a way of focusing on the individual experience (pp.16–24). It was important to examine carefully what each participant said and how they said it, then look at this objectively by bracketing out anything already known about the phenomena and then also from a contextual, worldly point of view. The interaction between participants and their shared dialogue whilst they played with the clay and created their clay sculptures, was also important to analyse.

Reliability and validity are considered differently in phenomenological studies, in that 'essential meaning, the sense of the empirical rather than facts' is emphasised (Quail & Peavy 1994, p.47). Giorgi (1989) suggests that within phenomenological research trustworthiness can be established through the presentation of a thorough and convincing investigation, and the presentation of worthwhile findings when measured against the original aims of the study.

Demonstrating methodological congruence, including 'rigorous and appropriate procedures' is also important (Pereira 2012, p.19).

Through using a phenomenological approach, the aim is for a fuller understanding of the participants' personal body image experiences, and the description of clay work as an intervention which addresses 'real', rather than 'assumed' needs. As well as providing detailed accounts of participants' lived experience, phenomenological studies enable researchers to make *tentative generalisations* from the cross-case analysis (Smith, Flowers & Larkin, 2009).

A Phenomenological Approach to Art Therapy and Clay Work

A growing number of art therapists have used a phenomenological approach in their research (e.g. Carr 2015, 2018; Rostron 2010; Tjasink 2010; Craig 2009;

Persons 2009) and others have supported its use within art therapy (e.g. Betensky 1995; Skaife 2001). As Skaife (2001) says, phenomenology can be used effectively within the many different art therapy approaches and is particularly useful when describing the relationship between 'seeing, making art, relating with others and "becoming" in a social context' and promotes a greater 'prominence for art in art therapy theory' (ibid. p.49).

A phenomenological approach to art therapy means that the therapist seeks to develop an *authentic* relationship with their clients, becoming a 'mutual subject' who remains 'authentically present while being aware that the space is for the other' (Tjasink 2010, p.78). An embodied and existential phenomenological approach to body image recognises the *central role of the body* in all aspects of consciousness, perception, and human experience (Merleau-Ponty 2002), and the recognition that a negative body image will impact on a person's 'entire' life/world.

A phenomenological approach to their creative work is often used instinctively by artists, writers, philosophers, and poets, as a way to '(re)unite them with the ground of their lived experience' (van Manen 1990, p.9). Phenomenology has been described as 'a primal telling', or a language that engages the 'voices' of artists, poets, musicians to 'sing the world' (Merleau-Ponty 1973, quoted in van Manen 1990, p.13).

Phenomenology can also be described as 'the attentive practice of thoughtfulness' or 'a caring attunement' (van Manen 1990, p.12; Heidegger 1962), when researching the *essence* of human experience, and encompasses a description of the *lifeworld* or *lived experience* of the participants (van Manen 1990, p.9). Artistic creations all employ ways to reduce phenomena to its essences (Carr 2015, 2018), and as such are compatible with a phenomenological study.

Importantly an existential and embodied phenomenological approach to art therapy recognises the centrality of the role of the body in all aspects of perception, consciousness, and human experience (Merleau-Ponty 2002).

Further Development of Themes: Continuing the Iterative Process

Writing this book has given us the opportunity to revisit the data and the subordinate/superordinate themes previously identified in order to carry out further analysis and refinement of the themes identified. This equates to further utilisation of the IPA 'hermeneutic circle', introducing new ways of thinking about the data and the development of new learning (Smith, Flowers & Larkin, 2009, p.28). The themes identified were grouped into three Major themes as follows:

Making Connections and Making Meaning through Stories of Body Image and Self-Identity

Metaphor and symbolism
Focusing on the psychological elements of body image

Abstract body image forms
Humour and liminality

Clay work as *Meaningful Play*

Defensive strategies, building walls, and covering over
Sensory properties of clay work
Anger and clay work as cathartic process
Revisioning body image with the use of clay for reflection
Dissociation from the body and missing body parts
Working with clay whilst discussing the internal and external elements of body image

The Impact of Mothers and Others on Body Image and Self-Identity

The critical mother, others, and self
Motherhood
Body-shame and guilt
Aging, the changing body, and feeling invisible
Sadness and loss
Self-compassion and acceptance
Shared humanity and experiences of womanhood

Revisiting the data has brought clarification and the development of new insights, enabling new learning and new meanings to be found. These themes will be discussed, compared, and developed within the following chapter.

10 Adding the Glaze

Finding Meaning and Healing through Metaphor and Symbolism

Although the aim of this study was not necessarily to find generalisations across the participants' accounts, in line with an IPA study, common themes were identified, and this chapter presents a synthesis of these themes and the new knowledge and implications they bring to the field. Revisiting the data from different perspectives and carrying out a further iterative cycle of analysis has brought further clarification, and enabled the development of three master themes that highlight new knowledge, as well as a new protocol for art therapy practice in this field, that can also be used in further research (itemised in Chapter 8.). Here we summarise the master themes and the major themes that support them.

Master Theme One: Making Connections and Making Meaning, Using Metaphor, and Symbolism to Tell Stories of Body Image

The importance of using metaphor and symbolism to explore body image has been demonstrated by this study, and whilst it was first thought that creating an abstract body image was in some way avoiding the issues, we found that those women who used it were able to go deeper and explore more of their issues than those who created a realistic representation.

For meaning to be found, there is a requirement for a story to be created around it and through its many layers, and this study has shown that it is metaphor and symbolism that allow meaningful patterns and connections to be made and a story to be told. Metaphor and symbolism are familiar, yet complex linguistic constructs used widely in everyday life that promote diverse and imaginative ways of thinking, and learning. Justine from Study One was able to draw a complex story out of her semi-abstract body image sculpture (see Figure 24 on p.77), describing the metaphor and symbolism she'd incorporated within her sculpture in great detail:

> "The image represents me – absorbing and caring. The smooth piece in the circle is me – the calm part that allows me to absorb and also to consider

my response and reflect. The curved wings around the hollow are me enfolding things in care. The pearl in the smooth part of the hollow is my husband . . ."

Justine

This study corroborates the findings by Carr (2015, 2018) that relating stories of self-identity (of which body image is a key component) to an empathic witness, is an important way of *knowing the self* and *being known*. When compared with literal content, talking in metaphor has been shown to be more emotionally engaging (Citron & Goldberg 2014). However, the use of metaphor and symbolism by Cynthia may have produced an emotional distancing effect, meaning she could safely embrace her issues in an abstract image, something that was less revealing, and less painful for her to see than a *realistic* image of herself.

The use of abstraction/or abstract elements within their body image sculptures by 9 out of 16 participants was something that happened intuitively; however, it served to add meaning and significance to their sculptures. Imaginative and metaphoric thinking was also used in order to construct a story around their clay image, that revealed personal meanings and significance around how they wanted to be seen. This study has therefore demonstrated that the use of metaphor, symbolism, and abstraction within clay work enabled a more in-depth search for self-knowledge and meaning.

An important factor when working with clients who express their body image through metaphor and symbolism is the requirement for the development of an intersubjective symbolic capacity or *metaphoric attunement* between the client and therapist and other group members. This is to ensure that a high level of understanding can be reached, and that the layers of meaning can be unravelled together. Neuroscience tells us that by 'joining the dots' and forming meaningful patterns and connections, a reward system is triggered in the brain to produce feel-good chemicals, meaning that 'a-ha' moments bring feelings of pleasure and satisfaction. This means that there is a level of enjoyment in discovering the layered meanings and complexity added to the sculptures through metaphor and symbolism, thereby mitigating painful feelings. We suggest that the women involved in the study also achieved a broadening of self-referential associative thinking (Shohamy & Wagner 2008), through the use of metaphor and symbolism within their sculptures, enabling the development of positive affect (Barr 2009).

One of the interesting aspects of the use of abstraction and metaphor within a body image sculpture is its ability to 'hold' dualities, such as hope and despair, therefore mitigating feelings of cognitive dissonance (Carr 2015, p.11). Instead, contradictory 'truths' are communicated in a direct and sensory way, enabling different aspects of body image to be explored simultaneously. In Study Two Cynthia described her abstract sculpture (see Figures 33 & 34 on p.92) as both a defensive 'fortress' with 'cuts' around the top to represent pain, and as a container for a 'candle', saying "When I seek that place now, it's more of a happier solitude than it was before." In this way Cynthia weaves a story around her body image representation, one that she eventually finds solace in, despite recognising it as a place of 'solitude'. This equates to a holding of dualities and 'metaphoric attunement' within her sculpture, a process of subtly changing its meaning, as the story unfolds (Carr 2015, p.212).

The beauty of metaphor and symbolism as a tool for studying body image, is the belief that our capacity to understand metaphorical thought is grounded in embodiment. Therefore it is only because we have bodies that we are able to understand such language. This leads on to an acknowledgement that our 'cognition' or ability to reason, is also grounded in our embodied experience; therefore Lakoff's description of 'embodied cognition' (Lakoff 2014, p.2) is pertinent to this study, demonstrating that abstract thought requires an embodied meaning (ibid. p.7). This highlights the importance of embodied metaphors within body image clay work, and the centrality of embodiment as an instrument of meaningfulness.

Whilst the question of meaning in a person's life is often linked to how full and 'worthwhile' it has been as opposed to 'empty and trivial' (Taylor 1989, p.42), it is perhaps the meaning in relationships and presence, and our ability to share humour and meaning, that offer a sense of ontological security and feelings of being-at-home within one's own body (Carr 2015, 2018).

Humour and Liminality

Humour involves the use of complex forms of metaphor and symbolism in order to understand things such as double innuendos and satire. Humour therefore requires a complex knowledge of linguistics and social context in order for it to be understood and appreciated. This complexity demonstrates that humour is an imaginative way of interacting with others, and something that can create a sense of connection, in order to laugh *with*, rather than *at* others.

Humour was expressed frequently between the participants attending the clay work sessions, with laughter often punctuating their narrative, which indicates they felt comfortable within a group of women of similar age and demographic. The humour expressed was also adaptive and brought a sense of perspective, as well as emotional distance to otherwise stressful topics. The humour was therefore an unconscious social construct by the group members to ensure they each felt comfortable and as a way to maintain the emotional equilibrium. The group cohesion was also helped by expressions of humour and laughter, as unconscious questions of "do you get it?" and also "do you get me?" were answered, demonstrating the importance of humour as a measure of *being known* (Carr 2018).

Humour was also used by participants within the individual sessions, which may have helped them manage experiences of liminality, as metaphor, symbolism, and humour can help describe a liminal space or feeling. Liminal experiences can be described as events or experiences that take us to a place that seems 'un-home-like', and usually include 'change', whether invited or not, so the menopause and the associated bodily changes may take a woman to a 'different place' in their lives, where letting go of fertility and a youthful body can be difficult for some to accept. This may indicate a reason why the menopause is called 'the change'. This, combined with other family changes, such as 'empty nest syndrome' as teenage children leave home, can cause women to feel that their bodies and their social situation have changed beyond recognition. This study suggests that feelings of liminality require a form, such as meaningful play within clay work, where ritual, symbolic expression, and ambiguity, can be explored and expressed.

Master Theme Two: Clay Work as *Meaningful Play*

We found that clay work used as *meaningful play* enabled participants to learn about themselves and develop feelings of *empowerment* and *motivation*. In Study Two the participants were able to use creative strategies to begin the process of replacing previously learned negative patterns of thinking and behaviour, with new positive ones that supported a positive body image.

Play enables a unique way of knowing, through active experimentation and learning, and this study corroborates Souter-Anderson's (2010, p.51) 'theory of contact' regarding clay work, as something that enables physical, emotional, and metaphorical contact, although we call this *meaningful play*, as this also includes the importance of finding or developing meaning through play. Meaningful play therefore encourages freedom of expression and fosters creativity and imagination, in order to increase the potential for empowerment, growth, and self-knowledge.

Meaningful play requires a sense of authenticity, of ownership of one's story and a return to a sense of belonging and insightful understanding. Each of the women who participated in the sessions engaged with the playful aspects of clay work in their own way, and actively contributed to the discussion around body image, demonstrating that clay work can aid reflection on body image from a psychological, emotional, or physical point of view.

Creating body image sculptures in clay engages with our human need to present ourselves visually to others, and Priscilla used her clay sculptures to highlight that which required attention in her relationship with her own body, enabling the expression of body image issues that had been previously hidden and avoided. We suggest that the kind of metaphoric understanding or body image stories possible within clay work are different to those found in narrative or other forms of artistic expression, in that during the session the three-dimensional plasticity of clay means it can be changed and modified, to create new stories and meanings.

Meaningful play requires an empathic witness, as we recognise meaning is located in the intersubjective space between the speaker and the listener.

Without the reflected testimony of a witness, knowing the self through being known becomes impossible, as Carel (2004) says:

> . . . meaning is not generated by the speaker, rather it is located intersubjectively, somewhere between the reception of the listener and the intention of the speaker. If there is no one to receive my speech I become mute. I cannot speak or make sense at all, not even to myself.
>
> (p.230)

Our findings correlate with those of Sholt & Gavron (2006), who say that three-dimensional objects created by clients in a therapeutic environment can themselves become a symbol and metaphor for the client's inner world and experience, with some of the participants using their imagination to revision their inner representations of body image, as well as their outer, physical representations. Therefore, we believe that clay work as meaningful play, used within the supportive framework of art therapy sessions, can be used by women to find personal acceptance and develop a balanced and positive view of their body-self as a 'whole' rather than as a collection of 'imperfect' parts.

Defensive Strategies, Building Walls, and Covering Over

One of the common themes talked about by participants and identified within their sculptures was the 'building of walls' and 'covering over', as defensive strategies. As Veronica says, "I couldn't do anything until I'd made a wall." This demonstrates the versatility of a three-dimensional material, and its ability to be manipulated into 'walls' as protective spaces for the participants to place their body image sculptures behind. The need for walls to 'hide' behind demonstrates how vulnerable some of the women felt, when asked to create their body image.

Building defensive structures may also indicate a need to protect themselves from feelings of shame, indicating that their body image is poor. This may also indicate a recognition that they have to protect themselves, in that mothers and others may have caused them pain or shame at some point in the past regarding their body image. This is also a recognition that those who should offer unconditional love may inadvertently cause pain and suffering around body image. The sense of betrayal this brings may also cause those who are hurt to lack trust in others, and to 'hide' and build up defences.

When talking about her sculpture Cynthia weaves a story that begins with it being a 'fortress' and a 'dead sort of thing' to eventually becoming 'more alive':

> "And also, it's a protection [. . .] it's protecting my own space, as well as being – or maybe instead of being a place to withdraw, it's actually a positive space where you can withdraw to or I can withdraw to when I want to, and bring in the things that I want to have there, rather than feel

> I *should* . . . or, you know, that kind of stuff. But it's also to do with nature. I think these marks, they make it – that they make this feel more like an organic thing, and it's something more alive, and something living rather than a, sort of, very, smooth, dead kind of thing. This one's more flowing and this is more living. The scratchy bit is more, more of a living thing, I think, more alive, so – and that's how I do feel."
>
> *Cynthia*

Veronica also talked about the need to make a 'protective space' before she could create her body image sculpture:

> "I felt really exposed doing it. I couldn't make . . . I couldn't . . . I thought, I'm not doing anything out of this clay, and then, once I'd made a protective space, I could make something inside that."
>
> *Veronica*

The theme of 'covering over' or 'covering up' either metaphorically or physically was also evident within the body image sculptures or stories, indicating again a sense of vulnerability and shame. However, the three-dimensionality of clay enabled the participants to build defences, that they could then see, enabling them to recognise their issues and recognise 'hiding' as a coping strategy. Being able to literally stand back and view their sculptures from different perspectives helped them recognise the defences they had put around themselves.

Sensory Properties of Clay Work

This study corroborates the findings of Cohen and Mills (1999), demonstrating that the unique properties of clay work can help reveal issues around a distorted body image and introduce it into conversation in a way that clients are able to tolerate. We found that the three-dimensional and sensory tactile qualities of natural clay created an atmosphere for significant reflection amongst the participants. However, we found a clear difference between participants describing their body image through narrative, and creating it visually, as specific kinds of metaphor and symbolism were utilised within the fabric of the sculptures that work in a different way to narrative and have a more immediate and direct impact on our senses (Freeland 2010, p.189). The body therefore becomes visible in clay work in a way that is simply not possible in a purely verbal narrative response.

We suggest that clay work creates a unique way of seeing and knowing the embodied self, and provides the opportunity to develop a new and healing relationship with one's body. As such this project corroborates Henley's (1991) suggestion that the malleable, plastic, nature of clay means it appears to possess 'a life and body of its own' (p.67), and is a multi-sensory experience involving the sense of: smell, vision, touch, sound, and space. This multi-sensory experience may enhance the emotional impact of exploring body image issues, however, importantly the use of metaphor and symbolism may mitigate this, by incorporating the making of connections and meaning, something that has been found to trigger feel-good chemicals in the brain (Shohamy & Wagner 2008).

The fragile and unpredictable nature of drying and firing clay could be considered one of clays negative aspects; however, its fragility can be used as an important metaphor for loss, imperfection, and death, as well as repair, renewal, and recovery. Also, the sensory playful nature of clay helped participants to 'get out of their heads' and 'into their bodies', something that was not always easy or pain free, but provided a flexible creative solution, and a kind of *embodied knowing*.

Anger and Clay Work as Cathartic Process

This study validates the view expressed by Carl Jung, that in giving a thought or feeling a visible shape, strong feelings can be safely brought to the fore, and a deeper understanding of issues related to the body can be found. Within clay work emotions can be played out safely in the physical making of the sculptures, making the process cathartic in nature, enabling actions such as cutting, stabbing, inscribing, as well as smoothing, shaping, and scraping to be carried out.

The cuts Cynthia made into her body image sculpture were an indication of the anger and shame she felt; they were also indicative of self-harm and self-rejection, and Cynthia confirms "it's about the 'ugly' parts of myself". As Cynthia continued to talk about her sculpture, she began to recognise that 'hiding' herself had been self-damaging, and considered changes she could make: "Letting them show more, or not feeling I've got to hide them, either my physical thing – either physical things from the outside, or my anger, for instance, because I think that's something that I've hidden."

Cynthia was able to draw a complex story out of her abstract body image sculpture in order to safely explore her pain and anger, and she spoke about letting the marks relating to anger and ugliness be seen, as she continued to scratch the marks onto the top, as well as the inside of her sculpture.

Revisioning Body Image with the Use of Clay for Reflection

Body image is only an 'image' of how we imagine our bodies to be, and neuroscience has shown that this image is often wrong, or distorted by the self and others; therefore this 'image' can be revisioned, to something more positive or compassionate, an image that does not necessarily equate to changing the body itself. The idea of *repair* or *redemption* was not the direct focus of this clay work intervention; rather the focus was on *transformation* through a process of *revisioning* (Carr 2015, 2017). This correlates with Carr's (2015) findings regarding the use of portraiture with people living with life-limiting illness, and indicates that through creating the clay body image sculptures, the women involved found new ways of *seeing* and *relating* to their bodies, which in turn produced new ways of *knowing* themselves (pp.232–233).

Creating their body image sculptures, whilst also reflecting on their personal body image stories, was an integral part of the process of revisioning. Handling the malleable, sensory material appeared to help participants focus on their body image whilst also becoming absorbed in the process of building, scraping, cutting, and smoothing the material.

When creating their own body image in clay, the forgiving nature of the material enabled the participants to experiment while cutting away, smoothing, reducing, and replacing parts of the body image sculpture. This was an empowering process, as Cynthia said: "I've just started realising I actually have the power to shape who I am." This was an important breakthrough for Cynthia, realising she had the 'power' to shape who she was, both physically by creating an image, and through revisioning her body image story. This demonstrates the importance of a creative response to trauma caused by body-shame, as the women felt empowered to revision their body image stories through their clay sculptures.

When reflecting on the first body image sculpture she had created, Priscilla recognised that her hips were exaggerated, meaning that when making her second image she was able to cut this down to something more realistic and the following dialogue outlines her process of cutting off, and sticking back, pieces of clay:

> "Yeah, and I suppose it's true. It's all true, but it's not to scale. Right, there you go. Possibly a better representation [pause]. Stick it here. Hey-ho, stick it here. Stick it – it's actually, you know – alright, I can use half of that clay [pause]. It's an instant weight-loss program, fantastic [pause]. Now, I don't know where to stop [pause]. That bit sticks out a lot more. That sticks out a bit there [pause]. Bit of a tummy going on [pause]. That'll do. There you go. I've lost an inch. Excellent."
>
> *Priscilla*

The process of adding and taking away, enabled Priscilla to work out physically a 'better representation' of her body image. Accepting that there's a 'bit of a tummy going on' and that it 'sticks out a bit there', indicates a process of 'feeling her way' around the body image, until it 'feels' familiar. The multimodal nature of vision also highlights embodiment, meaning that human eyes are not just instruments of vision, but can also be seen as 'hands' that touch and explore the visible (Gallese 2017, p.14), as in 'laying our hands or our eyes on something'.

Dissociation from the Body and Missing Body Parts

Dissociation or disconnecting from their body was identified as a coping mechanism utilised by some of the women in the study. As Priscilla says: "But I think the only way that I can carry on is by [. . .] disconnecting completely." Priscilla underlines this long-standing dissociation by saying "I don't look at myself in the mirror." Another participant who seemed to dissociate from her body was Linda, from Study One. She also reflected on her sculpture, saying: "Gosh, I don't even think I've got a body. . ." (see Figure 11 on p.59). If the first step of recovery is recognising that you have a problem, these admissions of dissociation can be seen as part of the healing process.

Neuroscience research has highlighted that some people retain a body image that is no longer current, as Nancy says: "I am not sure that my body matches up with who I think I am in my head, if that makes any sense." Nancy also recognises that she has used a form of dissociation by pretending that her weight was not an issue, saying: "Yeah, I think I've always had an issue with my weight [. . .] but I've always pretended that I didn't."

Missing body parts and an inability to 'see the body as a whole' were evident within the sculptures by Sarah, Linda, Jenny, Edina, and Eleanor. Some participants also included extra body parts, as in Sarah's 'three heads,' whilst others were missing their heads, e.g. Eleanor's sculpture, perhaps indicating feelings of disembodiment, or dissociation from their bodies. A number of the sculptures were also missing arms and legs, although this may have indicated a lack of clay sculpting skills, as well as an unconscious decision not to create them, perhaps suggesting vulnerability and a lack of autonomy.

Master Theme Three: The Impact of Mothers and Others on Body Image and Self-Identity

One of the significant themes emergent from this study, was the negative influence of participants' mothers' attitudes to their own and their daughter's body image. Therefore, this study corroborates the finding that mothers, carers, or significant others – people from whom unconditional love and care is expected – can undermine body image from a young age, often through thoughtless words or subliminal messaging. Mothers who show anxiety about their own weight and looks will raise daughters with similar body image concerns (Shenaar-Golan & Walter, 2015; Choate 2015), and this can also be passed down through the generations (Arroyo, Segrin & Andersen, 2017).

These negative messages can result in life-long negative body image beliefs and feelings of shame for the women concerned, and sadly, many women undertake painful and costly cosmetic surgery, in order to change their bodies to fit the 'cultural ideal', in the hope that it will make them feel better about themselves. Many women remain on 'diets' for significant periods of their lives in the hope of reducing their size to something more 'acceptable', only to binge eat to ward off depression and anxiety, and others may develop eating disorders, particularly if their mother or carer has an eating disorder.

Within this study there was often a subtleness in the way beliefs about body image were passed down the generations; however, the effect was anything but subtle, often causing deeply negative beliefs and consequences for the women involved. As Priscilla says, talking about her mother:

> "Yes, saying 'It's a shame you've got my shape', or whatever. But, even worse, predicting that I would look just like her . . ."
>
> *Priscilla*

Cynthia also remembers critical messages from her mother:

> "I was quite big . . . tall for my age and quite well-built. And my mum is little, so I felt like this big, clumsy . . . and she used to call me 'you great big whatsit' and stuff like that, and it all went in . . ."
>
> *Cynthia*

Nancy also talked of her mother's negative views of others, something that has influenced her own views of herself and others:

> "It's funny how I think I picked up most of my mum's ways of being when I was younger, because my mum is quite judgmental. And so, I remember, being in the car and she'd see a woman who was overweight and maybe her belly was hanging out of her top or whatever, and she'd be like, 'Oh, that's just – you just don't want to see that kind of thing . . .' So, I think my judgement was always based on what my mum, sort of said."

> "And [. . .] I, kind of said, 'Oh God, if I had that, I wouldn't wear that.' And that's . . . my mum! [laughs] God, yeah. No, that's my mother [laughter]. I can blame my mother for an awful lot . . ."
>
> *Nancy*

It was found that 'others', whether 'significant others' or 'non-significant others', were also a cause of historical negative body image beliefs, with negative events remembered in high detail, suggesting that these memories were traumatic, as neuroscientific studies have shown that traumatic memories are remembered more clearly. Priscilla described her feelings of mortification when going shopping with her grandmother, finding that her grandmother could find clothes that fitted perfectly, whereas nothing fitted Priscilla.

In Study One, Sarah created her body image as a 'smile on a stick' (see Figure 6 on p.54), explaining to the group that she was at the gym once when a man she didn't know approached her and told her bluntly that her body was unattractive. A thoughtless remark by another person, significant or not, can therefore cause remembered pain and trauma that stays with a person for the rest of their lives:

> ". . . there are negative voices that come from my childhood about my legs as well . . . from my brother."
>
> *Cynthia*

Priscilla vividly remembers a friend's younger brother making thoughtless, but no less cutting remarks, that live with her still:

> "I was going to stay with some friends, and [. . .] she had a younger brother [pause] who said to her . . . 'Hasn't she got huge hips. . . .'"
>
> *Priscilla*

These remarks are so painful because women see themselves not as they are, but how they imagine others see them – in comparison to the 'cultural ideal' of impossibly thin, and yet 'curvy' women. Always having to second-guess what others think of them and their body size/weight/shape, is a painful and exhausting way to live, as is constantly comparing the self with others. This causes feelings of humiliation, body-shame, of not feeling good enough, and engenders fears of rejection.

This study corroborates Fisher's (1990) findings that a positive mother–daughter relationship is of utmost importance in strengthening a healthy female body image, and is a call to women everywhere to break the cycle of historical negative body image, and provide a positive role model, so that their daughters can grow up appreciating and feeling comfortable in their own bodies.

Motherhood

Women in Western and many other cultures, have traditionally been encouraged to suppress and overlook their own needs in order to focus on nurturing others and this has also been used historically as a measure of their worth. Messages that reinforce this attitude are played out in relationships and the media. Unfortunately, the impact of this can often be depression and social isolation (Echenbaum & Orbach 1993; Ernst 1987).

Motherhood was one of the themes discussed by most of the participants in Study One. Helena talked about her concern regarding the effect of her own words on her 9-year-old daughter, saying she had in the past said to her daughter: "Oh, I hope you don't have [. . .] thunder thighs like mummy." Helena said that she has in the past said it without thinking, and is now concerned, saying "I wonder if a comment like that would actually stay with her, you know." This demonstrates an unexpected result of just one session exploring body image, where participants who were mothers (13 out of 16 were mothers), became aware, perhaps for the first time, of how their own words may impact on their children's body image.

Several of the participants created body image sculptures that featured themselves and their children, suggesting that their self-identity as a mother was indivisible for them from their body image. This may indicate the all-pervasive nature of motherhood, particularly whilst caring for young children. Sarah's body image featured three heads, that Sarah called "me, my mummy head, and my work head", whilst Sunny created a sculpture of herself and her three small children in a boat or container.

Body-Shame

Body-shame is a feeling of humiliation caused by comparing one's body size or shape to others and is therefore driven by competition and conformity, often leaving women feeling flawed, or not feeling 'good enough' and in need of fixing in order to be accepted by others. This study has shown that women drawn from the general population, who do not identify as having an eating disorder, still experience considerable feelings of shame around their body image, and as such fear humiliation, disconnection and abandonment by others. In order to find a way out of these endemic feelings of body-shame, an understanding of how girls in particular are parented, and how they are taught to look critically at themselves and others, needs to be developed. Within a society that is built on competition, comparison, and 'self-improvement', changing one's body image to avoid feelings of shame involves a process of swapping one's authenticity and uniqueness, for imitation, approval, and conformity.

Identifying shame and naming it is essential, so that women can develop a deep knowing that they are worthy of love, belonging, and respect, whatever size and shape they are. Priscilla relates a story here of body-shame, recognising that her unique body shape will not fit into off-the-peg clothes:

> "And then, one of my grandmothers wanted to take me shopping, and of course, you know, she could try stuff on and it all fitted, and there was nothing that actually fitted me. And it was just – it's almost humiliating, actually, that sort of thing. And it's not because anybody's saying anything, but it's just that fact that nothing really fits. So, it's actually quite limiting, I suppose . . ."
>
> *Priscilla*

Priscilla also talks about the shame she felt when having to go shopping with an uncle:

> "I went on holiday with my uncle and his family, and my suitcase got lost. So, it was one of those, I had to buy everything, and of course, actually buying things like swimming costumes and trousers is my worst nightmare. I hate shopping, and I had to go and do that with my uncle. And it was like, oh God, that's awful . . ."
>
> *Priscilla*

Nancy talks of avoiding body-shame by 'covering up' and wearing baggy tops:

> "And I'm more conscious of what I'm wearing, because I don't – the one thing I don't like is seeing rolls of [fat] [. . .] I would just be constantly trying to breathe in, or wear a baggy top. And that's it. I've been trying to wear more baggy tops so it [laughs] covers it up, and things like that."
>
> *Nancy*

This study has demonstrated that shame is a fear of disconnection, of being ostracised or found wanting, when comparing the self to others. Therefore, it is through building empathic connections to other women and allowing one's self to be authentically seen, that facilitates the development of self-compassion and the amelioration of feelings of body-shame.

Aging, the Changing Body, and Feeling Invisible

The effect of aging on the female body was discussed by the participants and featured in some of the body image sculptures. Cynthia said that her aging body brought with it a deeper consciousness of her mortality, but that this awareness had brought about a change of perspective, enabling her to consider "how I really want to live":

> "[. . .] I think it makes me more conscious of my mortality . . . and how I must live – my aging body and how I really want to live as best I can for myself now, and it's very positive. [. . .] I feel quite sad though, at the same time, because I feel I've – there's a lot of loss. And I feel – I think that the feeling is . . . *I've missed the bus* [laughter]. Just a waste, and I do feel sad about that, because of – I know there's no point in saying . . . in hindsight . . . 'Oh, if only,' – but I do fantasise quite a lot about if I had felt like this when I was 30, maybe."
>
> *Cynthia*

All the features that constitute the normalised ideal of female physical attractiveness in Western societies are those that belong to the young, fit, and fertile; none are associated with aging or the physical changes faced by older women. This means that aging can cause a decline in self-esteem and confidence and bring about feelings of invisibility, where they no longer feel validated by, or seen as worthwhile to, the wider community. Clearly women still care about their body image as they age, and often use cosmetics, plastic surgery, or other interventions to reduce the impact of aging. As long as appearance and conformity are the measure of a woman's value, the pressure to 'age gracefully' will be tantamount to remaining *young* (at least on the outside) for as long as possible. And the greatest compliment to an older woman will continue to be "you haven't aged a day since I last saw you . . ."

At the age of only 44 Jenny talks of feeling invisible, saying "I tend to think people don't see my face. I'm invisible now. I'm just a blob." However, many of the participants also talked about 'hiding' themselves; therefore a tension seems to exist between being seen and not seen, or perhaps, being seen on one's own terms is impossible for a woman, as she is always seen in relation to the cultural norms or ideals.

There were few perceived benefits with advancing years identified by the participants, however Cynthia identifies 'wisdom' as one, saying that she had traded her *youth* for *wisdom*. However, there is no suggestion that this is a trade-off she would have willingly made – rather it was one forced upon her by the relentless progress of time.

The Betrayal of the Body – Sadness, Pain, and Loss

The sculptures created by the women involved with the study became an embodiment of their body image stories, including pain, shame, anxiety, but also acceptance. Several of the participants created sculptures that embodied their feelings of sadness, pain, and loss around body image. Cynthia referred to her sculpture when she said:

> "It's pain. It's pain. It's something about pain, as well."
>
> *Cynthia*

Cynthia's 'pain' is perhaps an indication of the hurt and shame of all women who do not feel 'good enough,' or who are judged by their body shape or weight, rather than *who* or *what* they are. Cynthia explains her pain as

> "I felt sadness and almost tearful when I was scraping out a hollow within myself, my womb? My children? Abortions? Loss, not of use, my age, lack of sexual loving relationship, mourning old past relationships. Using my body, abusing, letting it be abused, I felt protective of what is left. The overflowing muffin hangover on my middle seems like a protective layer. Going through the menopause, a crossroads, ending – fear. I hate the spare part that flops over my jeans, like in the sculpture, trying to fit into something I've outgrown, wanting to fit into it. Not wanting to accept I've grown up."
>
> *Cynthia*

Victoria talked about feelings of loss regarding her 'athletic, healthy body', and her feelings of guilt at being unable to reverse this. Jane also spoke about regretting the loss of her once fit and athletic body, as did Jenny – saying she had once been slim and fit through running and going to the gym when she had first met her husband.

Jenny talked about how her husband had told her seven years earlier that she was 'unattractive' because of her size, something which added to her admitted 'hatred' of her body. Jenny also talked about an embodiment of sadness and loss, in that she had miscarried their baby and had been unable to conceive again, compounding her sadness and body-hatred, perhaps feeling it had let her down in her efforts to be a mother. Jenny then revealed to the group that she 'hated' her body and how this stopped her from enjoying trips with her husband to beautiful places in the world where he associates with beautiful people, preferring instead to stay at home where she wouldn't be judged.

Helena also spoke openly to the group about having experienced two late miscarriages, again emphasising sadness and loss around possible feelings of betrayal by the body. It is also interesting to note that her body image sculpture was constructed with an enlarged abdomen and therefore looked 'pregnant' (see Figure 4 on p.52). However, in her written reflections Helena described the group session she'd attended as 'compelling, emotional and gratifying', saying that the time spent creating her sculpture helped her realise that reflecting on her body image – although at times painful – had helped her come to terms with the losses she associated with her body image. This demonstrates that Helena felt even one group session of clay work was a therapeutic and healing experience.

Self-Compassion, Acceptance, and Shared Experiences of Womanhood

This study has shown that the development of self-compassion can be an important adaptive strategy for dealing with body image issues and feelings of shame. Whilst further research employing longitudinal studies is clearly required, drawing conclusions around this study offers an opportunity to begin the development of a theory of self-compassion in relation to body image and clay work. These tentative conclusions show that self-compassion and feelings of solidarity with other women can be developed through *clay work* that involves *meaningful play, metaphoric attunement* and being *authentically seen*, within a supported art therapy group, and in the presence of a trained art therapist. This corroborates Ferreira et al.'s view that body-shame can be ameliorated by the development of self-compassion, feelings of community, and acceptance through shared experiences of womanhood (2013, 2019).

Shame and humiliation equate to a fear of disconnection and feeling unworthy of love and attention, whilst being authentically seen involved accepting vulnerability, and allowing one's self to be seen without artifice or pretense. Research has also shown that women who find it difficult to be self-compassionate towards themselves often believe that others view them in a negative way (Ferreira et al. 2013, p.210). However, through sharing personal stories and experiences of body-shame within the group sessions, the women in this study were able to find a sense of solidarity and kinship, as they recognised their own issues were mirrored by other group members.

Within this study, the role of the art therapist/researcher as witness and safeguarder meant allowing the women to develop peer support and empathy for each other. We believe this was an important part of the process, and therefore group work, even if it is prior to individual work, is recommended. However, each client should be assessed on an individual basis to ensure that any therapy offered is right for them and their particular circumstances.

The stories of body image that the women developed through and around their body image sculptures offered important knowledge of the historical and contextual background to the issues they raised, often enabling them to identify the root causes of their issues. As so many of the women discussed issues emanating from their mothers, we suggest that the role of body image, shame, and the mother–daughter relationship would be a useful area for future study, as well as the role of clay work groups to build self-compassion and feelings of solidarity with other women. In Linda's "All Women" sculpture (see Figure 10 on p.58) there is a suggestion that 'all women' have issues of some degree about their bodies, and it was therefore a recognition of solidarity with 'all women'.

This study demonstrated that giving women the space and support to create and talk about their body image gave them 'permission' to tell stories they had hardly, if ever, voiced before. It is therefore through telling stories of body image to others that we learn about ourselves, identifying which part of those stories have been inherited and which part are authentic reflections of the self. Rejecting the distorted mirror that is historical body-shame, can make the difference between living out stories of body image that cause humiliation and pain, and taking ownership of our stories, in order to live out our own authentic story every day.

The clay work and meaningful play brought to the fore many unexpected and distinctive feelings from the participants, some of which were corroborated by individual participants and some that were corroborated by the whole group. As Cynthia says, it gave her the opportunity for empathic connection and to be authentically seen, by not shutting people out, recognising that she is finally "letting in" people to her world, which means also being let into their world:

> "[. . .] There are a lot, rather a lot. But it's, like, not just me. [. . .] The more I get to know people and the more I'm sharing with people, either patients or friends, I'm letting in other people – or I'm listening more to other people's things that aren't so nice."
>
> *Cynthia*

Allowing one's self to be vulnerably and authentically seen, is anxiety-provoking in the first instance. However, vulnerability is often the birthplace of creativity, innovation, and change.

This process of 'letting in' suggests that Cynthia was beginning to open up about her feelings, and developing feelings of solidarity with other women, as she listened to their own issues 'that aren't so nice'. This involved letting go of the idea that other women are 'perfect', and beginning to accept that most women have body image issues similar to hers. Therefore, the women in this study developed feelings of solidarity with other women in the group who had similar experiences, something that has been shown to ameliorate feelings of social isolation and loss.

Even in the short time they spent together, the majority of small groups attended by participants in Study One became supportive peer groups, based on equality and compassionate support, meaning the members felt of value to the group, experiencing 'inclusion, co-operation, and mutuality' (Herman 2018, pp.166–167). The acceptance and belonging found within the small groups were powerful ways to ameliorate feelings of shame and stigma that may have been held by participants for a long time (Herman & Schatzow, 1984). Humour and laughter were frequently used in the groups and individual sessions, and this study corroborates Fink and Walker's (1977) findings, demonstrating that more laughter and less embarrassment occur when people of equal status are present, and they feel less threatened. This study has therefore shown that humour is an important factor in ensuring group cohesion and understanding, as well as a tool for lightening the atmosphere or mitigating emotion.

Final Reflections

We believe that the sculptures and stories of body image related in this book demonstrate the power and value of clay work as a significant therapeutic tool for exploring body image in art therapy and other therapeutic disciplines. Although clay work in recent decades has remained largely unrecognised and under-used in art therapy practice, this study has shown how valuable and powerful a medium it can be for exploring body image issues with female clients, within a supportive therapeutic framework. Results from the analysis have suggested that the development of new meanings and learning about body image issues can be facilitated through *meaningful play*, providing a positive and contained opportunity for women to tell their stories through metaphor and symbolism.

The stories arising from the participants' body image sculptures have raised awareness of the underlying issues that many women face and the benefits they gained from the opportunity of working through their issues in a therapeutic environment. Body image and body self-esteem are a key aspect of a woman's sense of self-identity, and yet something that many of them dissociate from as a coping strategy. For these women, their bodies are a private source of shame and pain, something to be 'covered over' and hidden from view, not just from 'others' but from themselves, by avoiding mirrors or clothes that will reveal their shape.

During the group discussions it became evident that many of the women lived with both positive and negative body image views, most of which were rarely if ever articulated, instead remaining as a painful secret. However, the women who took part in the study were able to access deep and long-held beliefs and buried pain, and with the supportive process bring these out into the open to become *authentically seen.* This meant that the sessions were at times painful and at times angry, although a sense of humour prevailed as the women discovered how much they had in common, and the group members were able to offer each other empathy and support, in building each other's confidence, through the common bond of womanhood. This emphasises the positive function of group sessions for exploring body image issues, where peer support is a vital component towards developing self-compassion.

This study has shown that some stories we take on as our own, but they do not really belong to us – they are stories passed down by others when we are very young. These stories can become deeply ingrained and define who we think we are; indeed, we can carry around the psychological legacy of our mothers or others for the whole of our lives, both the good and the bad, unless we have the opportunity to confront, unpick, and *revision* these stories.

Although personal histories or hurtful incidents cannot be changed, the stories we tell ourselves and others can be. This builds on the belief that identifying the stories of body image that a person tells to themselves and others, and lives out every day, is an important first step to recognising where these stories originated from, and deciding if they originate from, or have been distorted by, other people's issues. This can help women to decide to take ownership of these stories or not, or to develop a new story of body image to tell themselves and others, that is based on self-compassion and self-love. A revisioned body image therefore includes recapturing one's self as valuable and lovable, and letting go of the need for perfectionism or conformity, in order to feel good about one's self, thereby breaking the cycle of shame.

We found that clay work within a group situation, with women of a similar age, enabled a process of intersubjective and embodied exploration of body image. For the women who used metaphor and symbolism within their sculptures there was a sense that they had begun a process of healing, moving their body image stories along and embracing clay work as a creative solution, leading to new ways of being and relating to the self and others, and a new flexible kind of *knowing.*

As we reflect on the completion of this study and the process of learning it has involved, we recognise that the development of solidarity and self-compassion around body image brings with it feelings of companionship and being valued, of 'fitting in' without the pain of judgement, and that it is within this supportive community that societal norms around body image can be challenged and ultimately overcome. This brings us back to the place we began this journey – with Trisha's *Army of Women* (see Figure 46 on p.178), joined together in companionship and solidarity, where the uniqueness of each individual is celebrated, and difference is prized over conformity and sameness . . . *which one are you?*

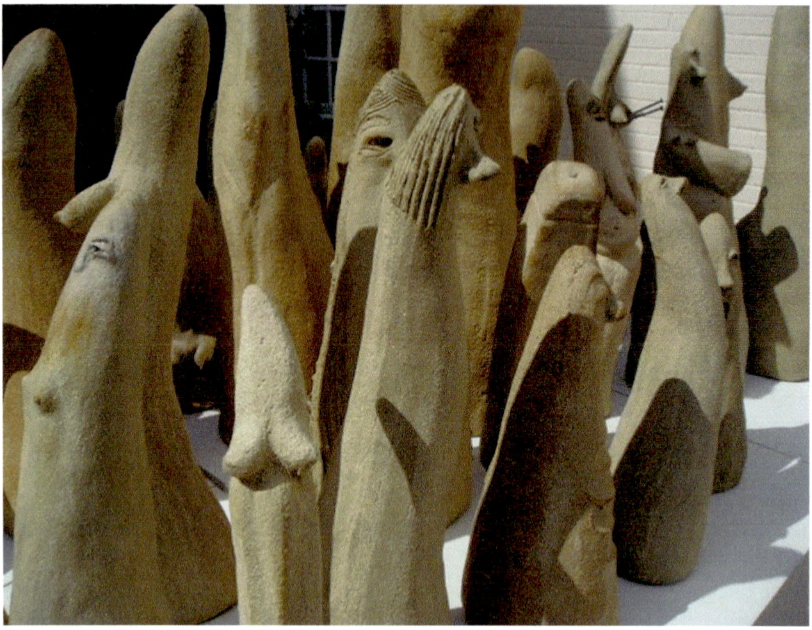

Figure 46 "An Army of Women No. 2" by Trisha Crocker.

Bibliography

Abramowitz, K. (2013) The unstructured use of clay in art therapy with older adults. *Canadian Art Therapy Association Journal*, Vol.26(1), pp.1–12.

Adamson E. (1970) 'Art for health' (pp.147–162). In, J. Creddy (Ed.) (1970) *The Social Context of Art*. London: Tavistock.

Adolphs, Ralph. (2004) Emotional vision. *Nature Neuroscience*, Vol.7, pp.1167–1168.

Akhtar, S. & Samuel, S. (1996) The concept of identity: Developmental origins, phenomenology, clinical relevance, and measurement. *Harvard Review of Psychiatry*, Vol.3(5), pp.254–267.

Alam, M. & Dover, J. (2001) On beauty: Evolution, psychosocial considerations, and surgical enhancement. *Arch. Dermatol.*, Vol.137, pp.795–807.

Anderson, A. & Phelps, E. (2001) Lesions of the human amygdala impair enhanced perception of emotionally salient events. *Nature*, Vol.411, pp.305–309.

Argyris, C. (1999) *On Organizational Learning* (2nd Ed.). Malden, MA: Blackwell.

Arroyo, A., Segrin, C. & Andersen, K. (2017) Intergenerational transmission of disordered eating: Direct and indirect maternal communication among grandmothers, mothers, and daughters. *Body Image*, Vol.20, pp.107–115.

Avison, D., Lau, F., Myers, M. & Nielsen, P. (1999) Action research. *Communications of ACM*, Vol.42(1), pp.94–97.

Bar, M. (2009) A cognitive neuroscience hypothesis of mood and depression. *Trends in Cognitive Science*, Vol.13, pp.456–463.

Battaglia, L & McNamara, B. (2012) Attachment styles and anorexia nervosa: A literature review. *Modern Psychological Studies*, Vol.17(2), pp.50–57.

Bauman, Z. (2004) *Identity: Conversations with Benedetto Vecchi.* Cambridge, UK & Malden, MA: Polity Press.

Baxter, L., Hughes, C. & Tight, M. (2001) *How to Research* (2nd Ed.). Buckingham: Open University Press.

Bedford, J. & Johnson, C. (2006) Societal influences on body image dissatisfaction in younger and older women. *Journal of Women and Aging*, Vol.18, pp.41–55.

Belfi, A., Vessel, E., Brielmann, A., Isik, A., Chatterjee, A., Leder, H., Pelli, D. & Starr, G. (2019) Dynamics of aesthetic experience are reflected in the default-mode network. *NeuroImage*, Vol.188, pp.584–597.

Berntsen, D. (2001) Involuntary memories of emotional events: Do memories of traumas and extremely happy events differ? *Applied Cognitive Psychology*, Vol.15(7), pp.135–158.

Betensky, M. (1995) *What Do You See? Phenomenology of Therapeutic Art Expression.* London: Jessica Kingsley.

Birmingham, C. & Treasure, J. (2010) *Medical Management of Eating Disorders*. New York: Cambridge University Press.

Bodner, R. & Prelec, D. (2002) 'Self-signaling and diagnostic utility in everyday decision making' (pp.105–126). In, I. Brocas & J. Carillo (Eds.) *The Psychology of Economic Decisions, Vol.1 Rationality and Well-Being*, Oxford: Oxford University Press.

Bradbury, H. (2008) 'Introduction: How to Situate and Define Action Research' (pp.1–12). In, P. Reason, and H. Bradbury (2008) (Eds.) *The Sage Handbook of Action Research: Participative Inquiry and Practice*. Thousand Oaks, CA: Sage.

Brock, M. (1991). The therapeutic use of clay. *British Journal of Occupational Therapy,* Vol.54(1), pp.13–15.

Brown, B. (2010) *The Gifts of Imperfection: Let Go of Who You Think You're Supposed to Be and Embrace Who You Are*. Center City, MN: Hazelden Publishing.

Brown, B. (2006) Shame Resilience Theory: A grounded theory study on women and shame, *Families in Society: The Journal of Contemporary Social Services*, Vol.87(1), pp.43–52.

Brown, S. & Vaughan, C. (2009) *Play: How It Shapes the Brain, Opens the Imagination, and Invigorates the Soul.* New York: Penguin Group.

Bruyneel, L., van Steenbergen, H., Hommel, B., Band, G., De Raedt, R. & Koster, E. (2013) Happy but still focused: failures to find evidence for a mood-induced widening of visual attention. *Psychological Research*, Vol.77, pp.320–332.

Bubl, E. et al. (2010) Seeing gray when feeling blue? Depression can be measured in the eye of the diseased. *Biological Psychiatry*, Vol.68(2), pp.205–208.

Buchalter, S. I. (2004) *A Practical Art Therapy.* London: Jessica Kingsley.

Buckner, R. & Carroll, D. (2006) Self-projection and the brain. *TRENDS in Cognitive Sciences*, Vol.11(2), pp.49–57.

Butler, J. (2006) [2004] *Precarious Life: The Powers of Mourning and Violence.* London & New York: Verso.

Calvo-Merino, B., Urgesi, C., Orgs, G., Aglioti, S. & Haggard, P. (2010) Extrastriate body area underlies aesthetic evaluation of body stimuli. *Experimental Brain Research*, Vol.204(3), pp.447–456.

Cameron, E., Ward, P., Mandville-Anstey, S., Coombs, A. (2019) The female aging body: A systematic review of female perspectives on aging, health, and body image. *Journal of Women Aging*, Vol.2:31(1), pp.3–17.

Cancienne, M. & Snowber, C. (2009) 'Writing rhythm: Movement as method' (pp.198–214). In, P. Leavy, *Method Meets Art: Arts-Based Research Practice* (pp.198–214). London & New York: Guilford Press.

Carel, H. (2008) *Illness: The Cry of the Flesh.* Stocksfield, UK: Acumen Publishing.

Carel, H. (2004) 'Philosophy as listening, the Lessons of Psychoanalysis' (pp.225–238). In, C. Havi & D. Gamez (Eds.) *What Philosophy IS*. London & New York: Continuum.

Carr, S. (2018) *Portrait Therapy: Resolving Self-Identity Disruption in Clients with Life-Threatening and Chronic Illnesses.* London & Philadelphia: Jessica Kingsley.

Carr, S. M. D. (2015) Enabling self-identity revisioning through portraiture, for people living with life threatening and chronic illnesses: 'Paint Me This Way!' *Loughborough University PhD Thesis.*

Carr, S. (2014) Revisioning self-identity: The role of portraits, neuroscience and the art therapist's 'third hand'. *The International Journal of Art Therapy*, Vol.19(2), pp.54–70.

Carr, S. & Hancock, S. (2017) Healing the inner child through portrait therapy: Illness, identity and childhood trauma. *International Journal of Art Therapy*, Vol.22(1), pp.8–21.

Case, C. & Dalley, T. (2000) *The Handbook of Art Therapy*. New York & Hove: Routledge.

Cash, T. (2004) Body image: Past, present, and future. *Body Image: An International Journal of Research,* Vol.1, pp.1–5.

Cash, T. (1990) 'The psychology of physical appearance: Aesthetics, attributes, and images' (pp.51–79). In, T. Cash & T. Pruzinsky (Eds.) *Body Images: Development, Deviance, and Change*. New York: Guilford Press.

Cash, T. & Pruzinsky, T. (Eds.) (2002a) 'Future challenges for Body Image Theory, Research, and Clinical Practice' (pp.509–516). In, T. Cash and T. Pruzinsky (Eds.) *Body-image: A Handbook of Theory, Research and Clinical Practice*. New York: Guilford Press.

Cash, T. & Pruzinsky, T. (Eds.) (2002b) *Body-image: A Handbook of Theory, Research and Clinical Practice*. New York: Guilford Press.

Cash, T. & Szymanski, M. (1995) Body-image disturbances and self-discrepancy theory: Expansion of the Body-Image Ideals Questionnaire. *Journal of Social and Clinical Psychology,* Vol.14(2), pp.134–146.

Cattaneo, Z. (2020) Neural correlates of visual aesthetic appreciation: insights from non-invasive brain simulation. *Experimental Brain Research*, Vol.283, pp.1–16.

Cattaneo, Z., Schiavi, S., Silvanto, J. & Nadal, M. (2017) A TMS study on the contribution of visual area V5 to the perception of implied motion in art and its appreciation. *Cognitive Neuroscience*, Vol.8(1), pp.59–68.

Cattaneo, Z., Lega, C., Ferrari, C., Vecchi, T., Cela-Conde, C., Silvanto, J. & Nadal, M. (2015) The role of the lateral occipital cortex in aesthetic appreciation of representational and abstract paintings: A TMS study. *Brain & Cognition*, Vol.95, pp.44–53.

Cazzato, V., Mele, S. & Urgesi, C. (2016) Different contributions of visual and motor brain areas during liking judgments of same-and-different-gender-bodies. *Brain Research,* Vol.1646, pp.98–108.

Cazzato, V., Mele, S. & Urgesi, C. (2014) Gender differences in the neural underpinning of perceiving and appreciating the beauty of the body. *Behavioural Brain Research*, Vol.264, pp.188–196.

Chatterjee, A & Vartanian, O. (2014) Neuroaesthetics. *Trends in Cognitive Science*, Vol.23(1), pp.53–62.

Chevalier, J. & Buckles, D. (2013) *Participatory Action Research: Theory and Methods for Engaged Inquiry*. London: Routledge.

Choate, L. (2015) *Swimming Upstream: Parenting Girls for Resilience in a Toxic Culture.* New York: Oxford University Press.

Citron, F. & Goldberg, A. (2014) Metaphorical sentences are more emotionally engaging than their literal counterparts. *Journal of Cognitive Neuroscience*, Vol.26(11), pp.2585–2595.

Clayton, J., Butow, P., Arnold, R. & Tattersall, H. (2005) Fostering coping and nurturing hope when discussing the future with terminally ill cancer patients and their caregivers. *Cancer*, Vol.103(9), pp.1965–1975.

Cohen, B. & Mills, A. (1999) 'Skin/Paper/Bark: Body-image, Trauma and The Diagnostic Drawing Series' (pp.203–221). In, G. Goodwin & R. Attias (Eds.) *Splintered Reflections: Images of the Body in Trauma*. New York: Perseus.

Cooley, E., Toray, T., Wang, M. & Valdez, N. (2008) Maternal effects on daughters' eating pathology and body image. *Eating Behaviors*, Vol.9(1), pp.52–61.

Coulson, S. & Lai, V. (2016) *The Metaphorical Brain*. Frontiers in Human Neuroscience, Vol.9. pp.1–3.

Cozolino, L. (2006) *The Neuroscience of Human Relationships*. New York: W. W. Norton & Co.

Craig, G. (2009) Intersubjectivity, phenomenology and multiple disabilities. *International Journal of Art Therapy*, Vol.14(2), pp.64–73.

Crocker, T. (2017) Me, myself and I: Women's perceptions of their body-image, using clay making as a tool for exploration. *PhD Thesis, University of Derby.* https://derby.openrepository.com/handle/10545/622774

Cula, G., Wu, I., Barkovic, S. & Appa, Y. (2010) Quantifying the effect of makeup on facial attractiveness. *Journal of the American Academy of Dermatology*, Vol.62, pp.1–10.

Daye, C., Webb, J. & Jafari, N. (2014) Exploring self-compassion as a refuge against recalling the body-related shaming of caregiver eating messages on dimensions of objectified body consciousness in college women. *Body Image*, Vol.11(4), pp.547–556.

De Morais, A., Dalécio, M., Vizmann, S., Bueno, V., Roecker, S., Salvagioni, D. & Eler, G. (2014) Effect on scores of depression and anxiety in psychiatric patients after clay work in a day hospital. *The Arts in Psychotherapy*, Vol.41, pp.205–210.

Delderfield, R. (2018) *Male Eating Disorders: Experiences of Food, Body and Self.* Cham, Switzerland: Palgrave Macmillan.

Descartes, R. (1996) [1641] 'Meditation VI' (pp.136–149). In, J. Cottingham (trans.) (1996) *Meditations on the First Philosophy*. Cambridge: Cambridge University Press.

Di Dio, C., Canessa, N., Cappa, S. & Rizzolatti, G. (2011) Specificity of esthetic experience for artworks: an FMRI study. *Frontiers in Human Neuroscience*, Vol.5(139), pp.1–14.

Dion, K., Berscheid, E. & Walster, E. (1972) What is beautiful is good. *Journal of Personality and Social Psychology,* Vol.24(3), pp.285–290.

Dissanayake, E. (1995) [1992] *Homo Aestheticus: Where Art Comes From and Why.* Seattle, WA: University of Washington Press.

Dissanayake, E. (1980) Art as a human behaviour: Toward an ethological view of art. *Journal of Aesthetics and Art Criticism*, Vol.38(4), pp.397–406.

Dupuis, A. & Thorns, D. (1998) Home, home ownership and the search for ontological security. *Sociological Review*, Vol.46, pp.24–47.

Ebner, N. (2008) Age of face matters: Age-group differences in ratings of young and old faces. *Behaviour Research Methods*, Vol.40, pp.130–136.

Echenbaum, L. & Orbach, S. (1993) 'Feminine subjectivity, counter-transference and the mother-daughter relationship' (pp.70–82). In J. van Mens-Verhulst, K. Schreurs, & L. Woertman (Eds.) (1993) *Daughtering and Mothering*. London: Routledge.

Edwards, D. (1999) The role of the case study in art therapy research. *The International Journal of Art Therapy*, Vol.4(1), pp.2–9.

Elbrecht, C. (2013) *Trauma Healing at the Clay Field: A Sensorimotor Art Therapy Approach*. London & Philadelphia: Jessica Kingsley.

Elbrecht, C. & Antcliff, L. R. (2014) Being touched through touch. Trauma treatment through haptic perception at the Clay Field: A sensorimotor art therapy. *International Journal of Art Therapy,* Vol.19(1), pp.19–30.

Ellis, M. (1989) Women: The mirage of the perfect image. *The Arts in Psychotherapy*, Vol.16, pp.263–276.

Epley, N. & Whitchurch, E. (2008) Mirror, mirror on the wall: Enhancement in self-recognition. *Personality and Social Psychology Bulletin*, Vol.34, pp.1159–1170.

Ernst, S. (1987) 'Can a daughter be a woman? Women's identity and psychological separation,' (pp.68–95). In, S. Ernst and M, Maguire (Eds.) *Living with the Sphinx*. London: The Women's Press.

Etcoff, N., Stock, S., Haley, L., Vickery, S. & House, D. (2011) Cosmetics as features of the extended human phenotype: Modulation of the perception of biologically important facial signals. *PLoS ONE*, pp.1–12.

Etherington, K. (2004a) *Becoming a Reflexive Researcher: Using Our Selves in Research.* London & Philadelphia: Jessica Kingsley.

Etherington, K. (2004b) Research methods: Reflexivities – roots, meanings, dilemmas. *Counselling and Psychotherapy Research: Linking Research with Practice*, Vol.4(2), pp.46–47.

Etherington, K. (2004c) Heuristic research as a vehicle for personal and professional development, *Counselling and Psychotherapy Research: Linking Research with Practice,* Vol.4(2), pp.48–63.

Evans, K. (2005) 'Body image and the construction of identity' (pp.38–49). In, D. Waller & C. Sibbett (Eds.) *Art Therapy and Cancer Care.* Maidenhead: Open University Press.

Fabre-Lewin, M. (1997) 'Liberation and the art of embodiment' (pp.115–124). In, S. Hogan (Ed.) *Feminist Approaches to Art Therapy*. London: Routledge.

Ferrari, C., Schiavi, S. & Cattaneo, Z. (2018) TMS over the superior temporal sulcus affects expressivity evaluation of portraits. *Cognitive, Affective, & Behavioural Neuroscience,* Vol.18(6), pp.1188–1197.

Ferraro, R., Muehlenkamp, J., Paintner, A., Wasson, K., Hager, T. & Hoverson, F. (2008) Aging, body image, and body shape. *The Journal of General Psychology*, Vol.135, pp.379–392.

Ferreira, C., Dias, B. & Oliveira, S. (2019) Behind women's body image-focused shame: Exploring the role of fears of compassion and self-criticism, *Eating Behaviors*, Vol.32, pp.12–17.

Ferreira, C., Pinto-Gouveia, J. & Duarte, C. (2013) Self-compassion in the face of shame and body image dissatisfaction: Implications for eating disorders. *Eating Behaviors*, Vol.14(2), pp.207–210.

Fesler, D., Nettle, D., Afshar, Y., Pinheiro Ide, A., Bolyanatz, A., Mulder, M.B., Cravalho, M., Delgado, T., Gruzd, B., Correia, M. et al. (2005) A cross-cultural investigation of the role of foot size in physical attractiveness. *Archives of Sexual Behaviour*, Vol.34, pp.267–276.

Festinger, L. (1962) Cognitive dissonance. *Scientific American*, Vol.207(4), pp.93–107.

Fink, B. & Matts, P. (2007) The effects of skin colour distribution and topography cues on the perception of female facial age and health. *Journal of the European Academy of Dermatology and Venereology*, Vol.22, pp.493–498.

Fink, E. & Walker, B. (1977) Humorous responses to embarrassment. *Psychological Reports*, Vol.40(2), pp.475–485.

Finlay, L. (2011) *Phenomenology for Therapists: Researching the Lived World.* Malden, MA, Oxford, Chichester: Wiley-Blackwell.

Finlay, L. (2009) Ambiguous encounters: A relational approach to phenomenological research. *Indo-Pacific Journal of Phenomenology*, Vol.9(1), pp.1–17.

Fisher, S. (1990). 'The evolution of psychological concepts about the body' (pp.3–20). In, T. Cash & T. Pruzinsky (Eds.) *Body Images: Development, Deviance, and Change*. New York: Guilford Press.

Fisher, S. & Cleveland, S. (1968) *Body-image and Personality*. New York: Dover.

Fonagy, P., Target, M., Gergely, G., Allen, J. & Bateman, A. (2003) The developmental roots of borderline personality disorder in early attachment relationships: A theory and some evidence. *Psychoanalytic Inquiry*, Vol.23, pp.412–459.

Foster, F. (1997) 'Fear of Three Dimensionality: Clay and Plasticine as Experimental Bodies' (pp.52–71). In, K. Killick & J. Shaverien (Eds.) *Art Psychotherapy and Psychosis*. London: Routledge.

Frank, A. (1997) *The Wounded Storyteller: Body, Illness and Ethics*. Chicago, IL: University of Chicago Press.

Franklin, M. (2010) Affect regulation, mirror neurons, and the third hand: Formulating mindful empathic art interventions. *Art Therapy: Journal of the American Art Therapy Association*, Vol.27(4), pp.160–167.

Frederickson, B. & Roberts, T. (1997) Objectification theory: Towards understanding woman's lived experience and mental health risks, *Psychology of Women Quarterly*, Vol.21, pp.173–206.

Freeland, C. (2010) *Portraits and Persons*. Oxford & New York: Oxford University Press.

Freud, S. (1913 [1899]) *The Interpretation of Dreams*. Stuttgart: Macmillan.

Fuller, P. (1980) *Art and Psychoanalysis*. London: Writers and Readers Cooperative.

Fuerstein (2009) *My Mother, My Mirror: Recognizing and Making the Most of Inherited Self-Images*. Oakland, CA: New Harbinger Publications.

Gadamer, H. (1975) *Truth and Method*. New York: Seabury Press.

Gallese, V. (2017) Visions of the body: Embodied simulation and aesthetic experience, *Humanities Futures*, pp.1–16.

Gallese, V. (2006) Intentional attunement: A neurophysiological perspective on social cognition and its disruption in autism. *Cognitive Brain Research*, Vol.1079, pp.15–24.

Gallese, V. (2005) Embodied simulation: From neurons to phenomenal experience. *Phenomenology Cognitive Science*, Vol.4, pp.23–48.

Gallese, V. & Lakoff, G. (2005) The brain's concepts: The role of the sensory-motor system in reason and language. *Cognitive Neuropsychology*, Vol.22(3–4), pp.455–479.

Gallese, V., Ferrari, P. & Umiltà, M. (2002) The mirror matching system: A shared manifold for intersubjectivity. *Behavioral and Brain Sciences,* Vol.25, pp.35–36.

Galmiche, M., Déchelotte, P., Lambert, G. & Tavolacci, M. (2019) Prevalence of eating disorders over the 2000–2018 period: A systematic literature review. *American Journal of Clinical Nutrition*, Vol.109, pp.1402–1413.

Gampel, Y. (1993) Access to the non-verbal through modelling in the psychoanalytic situation. *British Journal of Psychotherapy*, Vol.9(3), pp.280–290.

Gasper, K., & Clore, G. L. (2002) Attending to the big picture: Mood and global vs. local processing of visual information. *Psychological Science*, Vol.13(1), pp.34–40.

Gaudio, S., Dakanalis, A., Fariello, G. & Riva, G. (2018) 'Neuroscience, brain imaging, and body image in eating and weight eisorders: A guide to assessment, treatment, and prevention' (pp.97–107). In, M. Cuzzalaro & S. Fassino (Eds.) (2018) *Body Image, Eating, and Weight*. Cham, Switzerland: Springer.

Gaudio, S., Wiemerslage, L., Brooks, S. & Schiöth, H. (2016) A systematic review of resting-state functional-MRI studies in anorexia nervosa: Evidence for functional connectivity impairment in cognitive control and visuospatial and body-signal integration. *Neuroscience and Biobehavioural Reviews*, Vol.9(32), pp.578–589.

Gibbs, R., Costa, L. & Francozo, E. (2004) Metaphor is grounded in embodied experience. *Journal of Pragmatics*, Vol.36, pp.1189–1210.

Giddens, A. (1991) *Modernity and Self-Identity: Self and Society in the Late Modern Age*. Cambridge: Polity.

Giorgi, A. (1992) Description versus interpretation – competing alternative strategies for qualitative research. *Journal of Phenomenological Psychology*, Vol.23(2), pp.119–135.

Giorgi, A. (1989) Some theoretical and practical issues regarding the psychological phenomenological method. *The Saybrook Review*, Vol.7(2), pp.71–85.

Golomb, C. & McCormick, M. (1995) Sculpture: The development of three-dimensional representation in clay, *Visual Arts Research*, Vol.21(2), pp.35–50.

Gosselink, C. A., Cox, D., McClure, S. & De Jong, M. (2008) Ravishing or ravaged: women's relationships with women in the context of aging and Western beauty culture. *International Journal of Aging and Human Development*, Vol.66, pp.307–327.

Grogan, S. (2008) *Body-image: Understanding Body Dissatisfaction in Men, Women and Children* (2nd Ed.). New York: Routledge.

Grytten, N. & Måseide, P. (2006) "When I am together with them I feel more ill". The stigma of multiple sclerosis experienced in social relationships. *Chronic Illness*, Vol.2, pp.195–202.

Guardia, D., Cottencin, O., Thomas, P., Dodin, V. & Luyat, M. (2012) Spatial orientation constancy is impaired in anorexia nervosa. *Psychiatry Research*, Vol.195, pp.56–59.

Guegen, N. & Jacob, C. (2011) Enhanced female attractiveness with use of cosmetics and male tipping behavior in restaurants. *Journal of Cosmetic Science*, Vol.62, pp.283–290.

Gupta, M. & Gilchrest, B. (2005) Psychosocial aspects of aging skin. *Dermatologic Clinics*, Vol.23, pp.643–648.

Guseva, E. (2018) Bridging art therapy and neuroscience: Emotional expression and communication in an individual with late-stage Alzheimers, *Art Therapy: Journal of the American Association of Art Therapy*, Vol.35(3), pp.138–147.

Gussie Klorer, P. (2005) Expressive Therapy with Severely Maltreated Children: Neuroscience Contributions, *Art Therapy: Journal of the American Association of Art Therapy*, Vol.22(4), pp.213–220.

Halberstadt, J. (2007) 'Proximate and ultimate origins of a bias for prototypical faces' (pp.245–262). In, Forgas, J., Haselton, M. & von Hippel, W. (Eds.) (2007) *Evolution and the Social Mind.* Sydney: Psychology Press.

Hart, N. & Crawford-Wright, A. (1999) Research as therapy, therapy as research: Ethical dilemmas in new-paradigm research, *British Journal of Guidance & Counselling*, Vol.27(2), pp.205–214.

Hass-Cohen, N. (2008) 'Partnering of art therapy and neuroscience' (pp.21–42). In, Hass-Cohen, N. & Carr, R. (Eds.) (2008) *Art Therapy and Clinical Neuroscience*. London: Jessica Kingsley.

Hass-Cohen, N. & Carr, R. (Eds.) (2008) *Art Therapy and Clinical Neuroscience*. London & Philadelphia: Jessica Kingsley.

Hass-Cohen, N. & Clyde Findlay, J. (2009) Pain, attachment, and meaning making: Report on an art therapy relational neuroscience assessment protocol. *The Arts in Psychotherapy*, Vol.36, pp.175–184.

Hatch, M. & Yanow, D. (2008) Methodology by metaphor: Ways of seeing in painting and research, *Organization Studies,* Vol.29(1), p.23–44.

Hayes, G. (2012) Taking action in your research. *Interactions*, Vol.19(4), pp.50–53.

Heidegger, M. (1962 [1927]) *Being and Time*. New York: Harper & Row.

Hellema, P. (2011) 'She who laughs last . . .': The meaning of humour, as described by women in a creative arts process. *MIECAT MA Thesis*.

Henley, D. (1991) Facilitating the development of object relations through the use of clay in art therapy. *Art Therapy: Journal of the American Association of Art Therapy*, Vol.3, pp.67–73.

Henley, D. (2002) *Clayworks in Art Therapy: Plying the Sacred Circle.* Philadelphia: Jessica Kingsley.

Henn, M., Weinstein, M. & Foard, N. (2006) *A Short Introduction to Social Research*. London: Sage.

Herman, J. (2018) 'Shattered shame states and their repair' (pp.157–170). In, J. Yellin & K. White (Eds) (2018) [2012] *Shattered States: Disorganised Attachment and its Repair*. London & New York: Routledge.

Herman, J. & Schatzow, E. (1984) Time-limited group therapy for women with a history of incest. *International Journal of Group Psychotherapy,* Vol.34, pp.605–616.

Hill, S., Rodenheffer, C., Griskevicius, V., Durante, K. & White, A. (2012) Boosting beauty in an economic decline: Mating, spending, and the Lipstick Effect. *Journal of Personal and Social Psychology*, Vol.103, pp.275–291.

Hogan, S. (Ed.) (2003) *Gender Issues in Art Therapy.* London & Philadelphia: Jessica Kingsley.

Hogan, S. (2001) *Healing Arts: The History of Art Therapy*. London & Philadelphia: Jessica Kingsley.

Hogan, S. (Ed.) (1997) *Feminist Approaches to Art Therapy*. London & New York: Routledge.

Hogan, S. & Warren, L. (2012) Dealing with complexity in research findings: How do older women negotiate and challenge images of ageing? *Journal of Women and Ageing*, Vol.24(4), pp.329–350.

Holland, A. & Kensinger, E. (2010) Emotion and autobiographical memory. *Physics of Life Reviews*, Vol.7, pp.88–131.

Huang, M. (2009) The neuroscience of art. *Stanford Journal of Neuroscience*, Vol.II(1), pp.24–26.

Hughes, C. (2006) *Developing Reflexivity in Research*, University of Warwick: http://www.neuro-memento-mori.com/teaching/doc/research/developing-reflexivity-in-research.pdf

Hurd, L. (2000) Older women's body image and embodied experience: An exploration. *Journal of Women and Aging*, Issue 3–4, pp.77–97.

Hurd, L. & Griffin, M. (2008) Visible and invisible ageing: Beauty work as a response to ageism. *Ageing and Society*, Vol.28(5), pp.653–674.

Husserl, E. (1977 [1929]) *Cartesian Meditations: An Introduction to Phenomenology*. Nijhoff: The Hague (D. Cairns, Translation).

Husserl, E. (1970 [1954]) *The Crisis of European Sciences and Transcendental Phenomenology.* Evanston, IL: North Western University Press. (D. Carr, Translation).

Jaffe, K. & Worobey, J. (2006) Mothers' attitudes towards fat, weight and dieting in themselves and their children. *Body Image*, Vol.3, pp.113–120.

Jamrozik, A., McQuire, M., Cardillo, E. R. & Chatterjee, A. (2016). Metaphor: Bridging embodiment to abstraction. *Psychonomic Bulletin & Review*, Vol.23(4), pp.1080–1089.

Jokela, M. (2009) Physical attractiveness and reproductive success in humans: Evidence from the late 20th century United States. *Evolution Human Behavior*, Vol.30, pp.342–350.

Jolij, J & Meurs, M. (2011) Music Alters Visual Perception. *PLoS ONE* Vol.6(4), pp.1–7.

Jones, A., Porcheron, A. & Russell, R. (2018) Makeup changes the apparent size of facial features. *Psychology of Aesthetics, Creativity, and the Arts*, Vol.12, pp.359–368.

Jones, B., Hahn, A., Fishers, C., Wincenciak, J., Kendrik, M., Roberts, S., Little, A. & DeBruine, L. (2015) Facial colouration tracks changes in Women's Estradiol. *Psychoneuroendocrinology,* Vol.56, pp.29–34.

Jones, B., Little, A., Burt, D. & Perrett, D. (2004) When facial attractiveness is only skin deep. *Perception,* Vol.33, pp.569–576.

Jones, G. (2008) Visible mending: An enquiry into the experience of impermanence, imperfection and incompleteness. *MIECAT MA Thesis*.

Jones, M. (2003) 'From the peninsula: The geography of gender issues in art therapy' (pp.92–107). In, S. Hogan (Ed.) (2003) *Gender Issues in Art Therapy.* London & Philadelphia: Jessica Kingsley.

Jongeward, C. (2009) 'Visual portraits: Integrating artistic process into qualitative research' (pp.204–244). In, P. Leavy (2009) *Method Meets Art: Arts-Based Research Practice*. Guilford Press: London & New York.

Jung, C. (1933) *Modern Man in Search of a Soul*. London: Routledge.

Jung, C. (1916) [This publication 1960] 'The transcendent function' (pp.69–75). In, *The Structure and Dynamics of the Psyche*, Vol.8, London: Routledge & Kegan Paul.

Kagin, S. & Lusebrink, V. (1978) The expressive therapies continuum. *Art Psychotherapy,* Vol.5, pp.171–180.

Kelley, W., Macrae, C., Wyland, C, Caglar, S, Inati, S. & Heatherton, T. (2002) Finding the self? An event-related fMRI study. *Journal of Cognitive Neuroscience,* Vol.14(5), pp.785–794.

Keyes, M. F. (1984). The family clay sculpture in redecision therapy. *Transactional Analysis Journal,* Vol.14(1), pp.68–71.

Keysers, C., Wicker, B., Gazzola, V., Anton, J., Fogassi, L. & Gallese, V. (2004) A touching sight: SII/PV activation during the observation and experience of touch. *Neuron*, Vol.42, pp.336–346.

Kilpela, L., Becker, C., Wesley, N. & Steward, T. (2015) Body image in adult women: Moving beyond the younger years. *Advanced Eating Disorders*, Vol.3(2), pp.144–164.

King, J., Kaimal, G., Konopka, L., Belkofer, C. & E. Strang, C. (2019) Practical applications of neuroscience-informed art therapy, *Art Therapy: Journal of the American Association of Art Therapy*, Vol.36(3), pp.149–156.

Kirk, U., Skov, M., Hulme, O, Christensen, M. & Zeki, S. (2009) Modulation of aesthetic value by semantic context: An fMRI study. *NeuroImage,* Vol.44(3), pp.1125–1132.

Klein, M. (1952) 'Some theoretical conclusions regarding the emotional life of the infant.' In, M. Klein, P. Heimann, S. Isaacs & J. Riviere. (1952) *Developments in Psychoanalysis*. London: Hogarth.

Koren, L. (1998) *Wabi-Sabi for Artists, Designers, Poets & Philosophers*. Berkeley, CA: Stonebridge Press.

Korthase, K. & Trenholme, I. (1982) Perceived age and perceived physical attractiveness. *Perceptual and Motor Skills,* Vol.54, pp.1251–1258.
Kramer, E. (2000) 'The art therapist's third hand: Reflections on art, art therapy and society at large' (pp.47–72). In, A. Gerity. (Ed.) (2000) *Art as Therapy Collected Papers: Edith Kramer*. Jessica Kingsley: London & Philadelphia.
Kramer, E. (1977) Art therapy and play. *Art Therapy: Journal of the American Association of Art Therapy*, Vol.17(1), pp.3–11.
Kramer, E. (1971) *Art as Therapy with Children*. London: Schocken Books.
Kramer, E. & Schehr, J. (2000) 'An art therapy evaluation session for children' (pp.73–93). In, E. Kramer (1971) *Art as Therapy with Children*. London: Schocken Books.
Kwart, D., Foulsham, T. & Kingstone, A. (2012) Age and beauty are in the eye of the beholder. *Perception*, Vol.41, pp.925–938.
Lai, V., Howerton, O. & Desai, R. (2019) Concrete processing of action metaphors: Evidence from ERP. *Brain Research*, Vol.1714, pp.202–209.
Lakoff, G. (2014) Mapping the brain's metaphor circuitry: Metaphorical thought in everyday reason. *Frontiers in Human Neuroscience*, Vol.8, pp.1–14.
Lamb, C., Jackson, L., Cassiday, P. & Priest, D. (1993) Body figure preferences of men and women: a comparison of two generations. *Sex Roles*, Vol.28, pp.345–358.
Langlois, J., Rubenstein, A., Larson, A., Hallam, M. & Smoot, M. (2000) Maxim or myths of beauty? A meta-analytic and theoretical review. *Psychological Bulletin Journal*, Vol.126, pp.390–423.
Law Smith, M., Perrett, D., Jones, B., Cornwell, R., Moore, F. et al. (2005) Facial appearance is a cue to oestrogen levels in women. *Proceedings of the Royal Society* Vol.273, pp.135–140.
Lawler, S. (2008) *Identity: Sociological Perspectives.* Cambridge, UK, Malden, MA: Polity Press.
Leary, M. & Tangney, J. (Eds.) (2008) *Handbook of Self and Identity* (2nd Ed.). New York: Guilford Press.
Lesage, E. & Stein, E. (2016) Networks associated with reward. *Neuroscience in the 21st Century,* pp.1–27.
Levine & Smolak (2002) 'Body image development in adolescence' (pp.74–82). In, T. Cash and T. Pruzinsky, T. (Eds.) (2002) *Body-image, A Handbook of Theory, Research and Clinical Practice*. New York: Guilford Press.
Lewis, D. & Cachelin, F. (2001) Body image, body dissatisfaction, and eating attitudes in midlife and elderly women. *Eating Disorders*, Vol.9 (pp.29–39).
Liebmann, M. (1997) 'Art therapy and empowerment in a woman's self-help project' (pp.178–197). In, S. Hogan (Ed.) *Feminist Approaches to Art Therapy*. London & New York: Routledge.
Lusebrink, V. B. (2004) Art therapy and the brain: An attempt to understand the underlying processes of art expression in therapy. *Art Therapy: Journal of the American Art Therapy Association*, Vol.21(3), pp.125–135.
Malchiodi, C. (1998) *Art Therapy Sourcebook*. New York: McGraw Hill.
Mangweth-Matzek, B., Rupp, C., Hausmann, A., Assmayr, K., Mariacher, E., Kemmler, G. & Biebl, W. (2006) Never too old for eating disorders or body dissatisfaction: a community study of elderly women. *International Journal of Eating Disorders*. Vol.39(7), pp.583–586.

Marcus, B. (2004) Female passion and the matrix of mother, daughter and body: Vicissitudes of the maternal transference in the working through of sexual inhibitions. *Psychoanalytic Inquiry*, Vol.24(5), pp.680–712.

Martín-Loeches, M., Hernández-Tamames, J., Martín, A. & Urrutia, M. (2014) Beauty and ugliness in the bodies and faces of others: An fMRI study of person esthetic judgement. *Neuroscience*, Vol.277, pp.486–497.

Martin, W., Grey, M., Webber, T., Robinson, L., Hartt, N., Cairns, M & Stajduhar, K. (2007) Balancing dual roles in end-of-life research. *Canadian Oncology Nursing Journal*, Vol.17(3), pp.141–147.

Mauthner, N. & Doucet, A. (1998) 'Reflections on a voice-centred relational method of data analysis: Analysing maternal and domestic voices' (pp.119–146). In, J. Ribbens, and R. Edwards (Eds.) (1998) *Feminist Dilemmas in Qualitative Research: Private Lives and Public Texts*. London: Sage.

McBeth, A. & Gumley, A. (2012) Exploring compassion: A meta-analysis of the association between self-compassion and psychopathology. *Clinical Psychology Review*, Vol.32(6), pp.545–552.

Mciver, K. S. (2001) Spirit into form: The experience of clay as a spiritual practice. *Doctoral Dissertation, Colombia University, New York.*

McMains, S. & Kastner, S. (2011) Interactions of top-down and bottom-up mechanisms in human visual cortex. *The Journal of Neuroscience*, Vol.31(2), pp.587–597.

McNiff, S. (1992) *Art as Medicine: Creating a Therapy of the Imagination*. Shambala: Boston & London.

Medic, G., Wille, M. & Hemels, M. (2017) Short- and long-term health consequences of sleep disruption. *Nature and Science of Sleep*, Vol.9, pp.151–161.

Mellor, D., Fuller-Tyszkiewicz, M., McCabe, M. et al. (2010) Body image and self-esteem across age and gender: A short-term longitudinal study. *Sex Roles*, Vol.63, pp.672–681.

Merleau-Ponty, M. (2002 [1945]) *Phenomenology of Perception*. Routledge: London.

Mitchell, P. (1984). The role of regression in the treatment of depression with an intact ego. *Pratt Institute Creative Arts Therapy Review*, Vol.5, pp.17–21.

Moon, C. (Ed.) (2010) *Materials & Media in Art Therapy: Critical Understandings of Diverse Artistic Vocabularies.* New York & Hove: Routledge.

Morris, A. & Katzman, D. (2003) The impact of media on eating disorders in children and adolescents. *Paediatrics Child Health*, Vol.8(5), pp.287–289.

Munsteadt, K., Manthey, N., Sachsse, S. & Vahrson, H. (1997) Changes in self-concept and during alopecia induced cancer chemotherapy. *Support Care Cancer*, Vol.5, pp.139–143.

Nadal, M. & Skov, M. (2015) 'Neuroaesthetics' (pp.656–663). In, Smelser, N. & Baltes, P. (Eds.) (2015) *International Encyclopedia of the Social & Behavioral Sciences*, Vol.16, Oxford: Elsevier.

Neff, K. (2003) Self-compassion: An alternative conceptualization of a healthy attitude toward oneself. *Self and Identity* (2), pp.85–101.

Nightingale, F. (1992 [1860]) *Notes on Nursing: What It Is and What It Is Not.* London: Harrison & Son.

O'Brien, F. (2004) The making of mess in art therapy: Attachment, trauma and the brain. *The International Journal of Art Therapy*, Vol.9(1), pp.2–13.

O'Flynn, D. (2011) Art as healing: Edward Adamson. *Raw Vision*, Vol.72, Spring, pp.46–53.

O'Neill, M. (2008) Transnational refugees: The transformative role of art? *Forum: Qualitative Social Research,* Vol.9(2), Art, 59, pp.1–22.
Ochsner, K., Ray, R., Hughes, B., McRae, K., Cooper, J., Weber, J., Gabrieli, J. & Gross, J. (2009) Bottom-up and top-down processes in emotion generation: Common and distinct neural mechanisms. *Psychological Science*, Vol.20, pp.1322–1331.
Ogden, T. H. (1989) *The Primitive Edge of Experience.* Northvale, NJ: Jason Aronson.
Orbach, S. (1997) 'Women's development in the family' (pp.36–54). In, M. Lawrence & M. Maguire (1997) *Psychotherapy with Women: Feminist Perspectives*. London & Basingstoke: Macmillan.
Oyserman, D., Elmore, K. & Smith, G. (2012) 'Self, self-concept, and identity' (p. 69–104). In, M. Leary & J. Tangney (Eds.) *Handbook of Self and Identity* (2nd Ed.). New York: Guilford Press.
Palmer, P. (2007 [1998]) *The Courage to Teach: Exploring the Inner Landscape of a Teacher's Life*. San Francisco: Jossey-Bass.
Pascual-Leone, A., Amedi, A., Fregni, F. & Merabet, L. (2005) The plastic human brain cortex. *Annual Review of Neuroscience*, Vol.28, pp.337–401.
Pausé, C. (2007) Invisible women: Exploring weight identity in morbidly obese women. *PhD Dissertation, Texas Tech University, USA*.
Pelowski, M., Markey, P., Forster, M., Gerger, G. & Leder, H. (2017) Move me, astonish me . . . delight my eyes and brain: The Vienna integrated model of top-down and bottom-up processes in art perception (VIMAP) and corresponding affective, evaluative, and neurophysiological correlates. *Physics of Life Reviews*, Vol.21, pp.80–125.
Pereira, H. (2012) Rigor in phenomenological research: Reflections of a novice nurse researcher. *Nurse Researcher*, Vol.19(3), pp.16–19.
Perry, B. (2009) Examining child maltreatment through a neuro-developmental lens: Clinical applications of the Neurosequential Model of Therapeutics, *Journal of Loss and Trauma: International Perspectives on Stress & Coping*, Vol.14(4), pp.240–255.
Persons, R. (2009) Art therapy with serious juvenile offenders: A phenomenological analysis. *International Journal of Offender Therapy and Comparative Criminology*, Vol.53, pp.433–453.
Philips, J., Conheim, C. & Forester, C. (2000) *A Waist Is a Terrible Thing to Mind: A Wake-up Call*. California: Breakthrough Press.
Pietkiewicz, I. & Smith, J. (2014) A practical guide to using Interpretative Phenomenological Analysis in qualitative research psychology. *Psychological Journal*, January, pp.7–14.
Pink, S. (2004) 'Performance, self-representation and narrative: Interviewing with video' (pp.61–77). In, C. Pole (Ed.) *Seeing is Believing? Approaches to Visual Research, Studies in Qualitative Methodology*, Vol.7, Oxford: Elsevier JAI.
Pink, S. (2007) *Doing Visual Ethnography*. London: Sage.
Pinkola Estes, C. (1992) *Women who Run with the Wolves*. London: Random House.
Pointon, M. (2013) *Portrayal and the Search for Identity*. London: Reaktion Books.
Pulcu, E., Lythe, K., Elliott, E., Green, S., Moll, J., Deakin, J. & Zahn, R. (2014) Increased amygdala response to shame in remitted major depressive disorder. *PLOS One*, Vol.9(1), pp.1–15.
Quail, J. M & Peavy, V. (1994) A phenomenologic research study of a client's experience of art therapy. *The Arts in Psychotherapy*, Vol.21(1), pp.45–57.
Rabinor, J. & Bilich, M. (2002) 'Experiential approaches to changing body-image' (pp.469–477). In, T. Cash and T. Pruzinsky (Eds.) (2002) *Body-image, A Handbook of Theory, Research and Clinical Practice*. New York: Guilford Press.

Ramachandran, V. & Hirstein, W. (1999) The science of art: A neurological theory of aesthetic experience. *Journal of Consciousness Studies*, Vol.6(6–7), pp.15–51.

Ramsey, J., Langlois, J, Hoss, R., Rubenstein, A. & Griffin, A. (2004) Origins of a stereotype: Categorization of facial attractiveness by 6-month-old infants. *Developmental Science*, Vol.7, pp.201–211.

Reason, P. and Bradbury, H. (2008) (Eds.) *The Sage Handbook of Action Research: Participative Inquiry and Practice*. Thousand Oaks, CA: Sage.

Rhodes, M. (2008) 'Getting the inside out: Speaking with clay' (pp.27–45). In, D. McCarthy (Ed) (2008) *Speaking about the Unspeakable: Non-Verbal Methods and Experiences in Therapy with Children*. London: Jessica Kingsley.

Riener, C., Stefanucci, J., Proffitt, D. & Clore, G. (2011) An effect of mood on the perception of geographical slant. *Cognition and Emotion*, Vol.25, pp.174–182.

Riva, G. (2010) Neuroscience and eating disorders: The role of the medial-temporal lobe. *Nature Proceedings*, 24th February 2010, pp.1–8.

Riva, G. & Gaudio, S. (2018) Locked to a wrong body: Eating disorders as the outcome of a primary disturbance in multisensory body integration. *Consciousness and Cognition*, Vol.59, pp.57–59.

Rizzolatti, G., Fadiga, L., Gallese, V. & Fogassi, L. (1996) Premotor cortex and the recognition of motor actions. *Cognitive Brain Research*, Vol.3(2), pp.131–141.

Robbins, A. (1999) Chaos as form. *Art Therapy: Journal of the American Art Therapy Association*, Vol.16(3), pp.121–131.

Robbins, A. (1987) *The Artist as Therapist*. New York: Human Sciences Press.

Rogers, C. (2003 [1951]) *Client-Centred Therapy: Its Current Practice, Implications, and Theory.* London: Constable.

Rostron, J. (2010) On amodal perception and language in art therapy with autism. *International Journal of Art Therapy*, Vol.15(1), pp.36–49.

Rowe, G., Hirsh, J. & Anderson, A. (2007) Positive affect increases the breadth of attentional selection. *PNAS*, pp.383–388.

Roy, M. & Payette H. (2012) The body image construct among Western seniors: A systematic review of the literature. *Archives of Gerontology and Geriatrics*, Vol.55(1), pp.505–521.

Rubenstein, A., Langlois, J. & Roggman, L. (2002) 'What makes a face attractive and why?' (pp.1–33). In, G. Rhodes & L. Zebrowitz (Eds.) (2002) *Facial Attractiveness: Evolutionary, Cognitive and Social Perspectives* (Advances in Visual Cognition volume 1). Westport, CT: Ablex.

Rubin, J. (Ed.) (2001) *Approaches to Art Therapy: Theory and Technique* (2nd Ed.). Brunner-Routledge: New York & London, pp.178–188.

Rubin, J. A. (1984) *Child Art Therapy: Understanding and Helping Children Grow through Art* (2nd Ed.). New York: Van Nostrand Reinhold.

Russell, R., Sweda, J., Porcheron, A. & Mauger E. (2014) Sclera colour changes with age and is a cue for perceiving age, health, and beauty. *Psychology and Aging*, Vol.29, pp.626–635.

Russell, R., Batres, C., Courreges, S., Kaminski, G., Soppelsa, F. et al. (2018) Differential effects of makeup on perceived age. *British Journal of Psychology*, Vol.110(1), pp.87–100.

Samino, E. (2010) Descriptions of pain, metaphor and embodied simulation. *Metaphor and Symbol*, Vol.25(4), pp.205–226.

Samson, N., Fink, B. & Matts, P. (2010) Visible skin condition and perception of human facial appearance. *International Journal of Cosmetic Science*, Vol.32, pp.167–184.

Schaverien, J. (2000) 'The triangular relationship and the aesthetic countertransference in analytical art psychotherapy' (pp.55–83). In, A. Gilroy & G. McNelly (Eds.) (2000) *The Changing Shape of Art Therapy: New Developments in Theory and Practice.* London: Jessica Kingsley.

Schilder, P. (1950) *The Image and Appearance of the Human Body.* New York & London: Routledge.

Schlossberg, I. (1983) The ego organising qualities of various media in an acute psychiatric population. *Pratt Creative Arts Review*, Vol.4, pp.22–28.

Schwartz, M. & Brownell, K. (2002) 'Obesity and body-image' (pp.200–209). In, T. Cash & T. Pruzinsky (Eds.) *Body-image, A Handbook of Theory, Research and Clinical Practice,* New York: Guilford Press.

Scruton, R. (2009) *Why Beauty Matters*. BBC Documentary, November 2009.

Seftel, L. (1987) A conversation with Edward Adamson. *Art Therapy, Journal of the American Art Therapy Association*, Vol.26, November, pp.48–51.

Shen, L. (2018) The evolution of shame and guilt, *PLOS One*, July, pp.1–11.

Shenaar-Golan, V. & Walter, O. (2015) Mother-daughter relationship and daughter's body image, *Health*, Vol.7, pp.547–559.

Shepperd, J., Carroll, P, Grace, J. & Terry, M. (2002) Exploring the Causes of Comparative Optimism. *Psychologica Belgica*, Vol.42, pp.65–98.

Shermer, M. (2004) *The Science of Good and Evil.* New York: Henry Holt & Co.

Sherwood, P. (2004) *The Healing Art of Clay Therapy*. Melbourne: Acer Press.

Shohamy, D & Wagner, A. (2008) Integrating memories in the human brain: Hippocampal-midbrain encoding of overlapping events. *Neuron*, Vol.60, pp.378–389.

Sholt, M. & Gavron, T. (2006) Therapeutic qualities of clay work in art therapy and psychotherapy: A review. *Art Therapy, Journal of the American Art Therapy Association*, 23(2), pp.66–72.

Sibbett, C. (2005) 'Liminal embodiment: embodied and sensory experience in cancer care and art therapy' (pp.50–81). In, D. Waller, Diane. & C. Sibbett (Eds.) (2005) *Facing Death: Art Therapy and Cancer Care.* Maidenhead: Open University Press.

Sinai, M., Ooi, T. & He, Z. (1998) Terrain influences the accurate judgment of distance. *Nature*, Vol.395, pp.497–500.

Skaife, S. (2001) Making visible: Art therapy and intersubjectivity. *Inscape, International Journal of Art Therapy*, Vol.6(2), pp.40–50.

Skaife, S. (2000) 'Keeping the balance. Further thoughts on the dialectics of art therapy' (pp.115–142). In, A. Gilroy & G. McNeilly (Eds.) *The Changing Shape of Art Therapy*. London & Philadelphia: Jessica Kingsley.

Skaife, S. & Huet, V. (Eds.) (1998) *Between Words and Pictures: Art Psychotherapy Groups.* London: Routledge.

SLaM (South London and Maudsley NHS Foundation Trust) (2018) *The Adamson Collection.*

Smith, J., Flowers, P. & Larkin, M. (2009) *Interpretative Phenomenological Analysis: Theory, Method and Research.* Thousand Oaks, CA, New York & India: Sage Publications.

Smith, J., Harré, R. & Van Langenhove, L. (1995). Idiography (pp.56–69). In, J. Smith., R. Harré & L. Van Langenhove (Eds.) *Rethinking Psychology*. London: Sage.

Snir, S. & Regev, D. (2013) A dialog with five art materials: Creators share their art making experiences. *The Arts in Psychotherapy*, Vol.40 (1) pp.94–100.

Souter-Anderson, L. (2010) *Touching Clay, Touching What?* Dorset, UK: Archive Publishing.

Stefanucci, J. & Storbeck, J. (2009) Don't look down: emotional arousal elevates height perception. *The Journal of Experimental Psychology: General*, Vol.138, pp.131–145.

Stern, D. (1985) *The Interpersonal World of the Infant.* New York: Basic Books.

Striegel-Moore & Franko (2002) Body image issues among girls and women (pp.183–191). In, T. Cash, T. & T. Pruzinsky (Eds.) *Body-image, A Handbook of Theory, Research and Clinical Practice*. New York: Guilford Press.

Svenaeus, F. (2011) Illness as unhomelike being-in-the-world: Heidegger and the phenomenology of medicine. *Medicine Health Care and Philosophy*, Vol.14, pp.333–343.

Swanson, H., Power, K., Collin, P., Deas, S., Paterson, G., Grierson, D. et al. (2009) The relationship between parental bonding, social problem solving and eating pathology in an anorexic inpatient sample. *European Eating Disorders Review*, Vol.18(1), pp.22–32.

Sznycer, D., Tooby, J., Cosmides, L., Porat, R., Shalvi, S. & Halperin, E. (2016) Shame closely tracks the threat of devaluation by others, even across cultures. *PNAS,* Vol.113 (10), pp.2625–2630.

Tangney, J., Stuewig, J. & Mashek, D. (2006) Moral emotions and moral behavior. *Annual Review of Psychology*, (58), pp.345–372.

Tantleef-Dunn, S. & Gokee, J. (2002) Interpersonal influences on body-image. *The Arts in Psychotherapy*, Vol.22(5), pp.413–427.

Tatarunaite, E., Playle, R., Hood, K, Shaw, W. & Richmond, S. (2005) Facial attractiveness: A longitudinal study. *American Journal of Orthodontics and Dentofacial Orthopaedics,* Vol.127, pp.676–682.

Taylor, C. (1989) *Sources of the Self: The Making of Modern Identity.* Cambridge: Cambridge University Press.

Taylor, J. (2009) 'Proprioception' (p.1143–1149). In, L. Squire (Ed.) *Encyclopedia of Neuroscience*. London, Burlington MA, San Diego CA: Academic Press.

Tchkonia, T., Morbeck, D., Von Zglinicki, T., Van Deursen, J., Lustgarten, J., Scrable, H. & Kirkland, J. (2010) Fat tissue, aging, and cellular senescence. *Aging Cell*, Vol.9(5), pp.667–684.

Thone, R. R. (1992) Women and aging: Celebrating ourselves. New York: Haworth Press.

Thornhill, R. & Gangestad, S. (2008) *The Evolutionary Biology of Human Female Sexuality*, Oxford: Oxford University Press.

Tiggemann, M. & Lynch, J. (2001) Body image across the life span in adult women: the role of self-objectification. *Developmental Psychology*, Vol.37, pp.243–253.

Tjasink, M. (2010) Art psychotherapy in medical oncology: A search for meaning. *International Journal of Art Therapy*, Vol.15(2): pp.75–83.

Trevarthen, C. (2005) 'Stepping away from the mirror: pride and shame in adventures of companionship: reflections on the nature and emotional needs of infant intersubjectivity' (pp.55–84). In: C. Carter, L. Ahnert, K. Grossmann, S. Hardy, M. Lamb, S. Porges & N. Sachser (Eds.) *The 92nd Dahlem Workshop Report: Attachment and Bonding: A New Synthesis*. Cambridge, MA: MIT Press.

Trivers, R. (2002) Self-deception in service of deceit. In, *Natural Selection and Social Theory: Selected Papers of Robert Trivers*. Oxford: Oxford University Press, pp.255–293.

Turner, V. (1995 [1969]) *The Ritual Process: Structure and Anti-Structure*. New York: Aldine de Gruyter.

Turner, V. (1982) From ritual to theatre: The human seriousness of play. New York: Performing Arts Journal Publications.

Ueda, S. & Koyama, T. (2010) Influence of make-up on facial recognition. *Perception,* Vol.39, pp.260–264.

Ussher, J. (1993) *The Psychology of the Female Body*. London: Routledge.

van Gennep, A. (1960) *The Rites of Passage.* Chicago, IL: University of Chicago Press.

van Manen, M. (1990) *Researching Lived Experience*. Ontario, Canada: State University of New York Press.

Vecchi, B. (2004) 'Introduction' (pp.1–8). In, B. Zygmunt. (2004) *Identity: Conversations with Benedetto Vecchi.* Cambridge, UK & Malden, MA: Polity Press.

Vessel, E., Starr, G. & Rubin, N. (2012) The brain on art: intense aesthetic experience activates the default mode network. *Frontiers in Human Neuroscience*, Vol.6(66), pp.1–10.

Vessel, E., Isik, A., Belfi, A., Stahl, J. & Starr, G. (2019) The default-mode network represents aesthetic appeal that generalizes across visual domains. *Proceedings of the National Academy of Sciences (PNAS) USA,* Vol.116(38), pp.19155–19164.

Waldman, J. (1999) Breaking the mould: A woman's psychosocial and artistic journey with clay. *International Journal of Art Therapy*, Vol.4(1), pp.10–19.

Wallin, D. (2007) *Attachment in Psychotherapy*. New York: Guilford Press.

Weisfeld, G. (1993) The adaptive value of humor and laughter. *Ethology and Sociobiology*, Vol.14(2), pp.141–169.

Willig, C. (2010) *Introducing Qualitative Research in Psychology*. Maidenhead: Open University Press.

Wilson, F. (1998). *The Hand*. New York: Vintage.

Winnicott, D. (1975 [1950–5]) *Through Paediatrics to Psychoanalysis: Collected Papers* (2nd Ed.). Reprint. London: Karnac, pp.1–350.

Winnicott, D. (1971a) *Playing and Reality*. London: Tavistock.

Winnicott, D. (1971b) 'Mirror-role of the mother and family in child development' (pp.111–118). In, D. Winnicott (1971) *Playing and Reality*. London: Tavistock.

Winnicott, D. (1968) Playing: Its theoretical status in the clinical situation. *International Journal of Psychoanalysis*, Vol.50, pp.711–716.

Winnicott, D. (1960) *Ego Distortion in Terms of True and False Self. The Maturational Process and the Facilitating Environment: Studies in the Theory of Emotional Development*. New York: International Universities Press, pp.140–157.

Winnicott, D. (1953) Transitional objects and transitional phenomena: A study of the first not-me possession. *International Journal of Psycho-Analysis*, Vol.34, pp.89–97.

Woltmann, A. (1993) 'Mud and clay' (pp. 141–157). In, C. Schaefer & D. Cangelosi (Eds.). *Play therapy techniques.* Northvale, NJ: Jason Aronson.

Wright, K. (2009) *Mirroring and Attunement: Self-Realisation in Psychoanalysis and Art.* London & New York: Routledge.

Yarosh, D. (2019a) Perception and deception: Human beauty and the brain. *Behavioral Science* [special issue – Consumer Neurosciences], Vol.9(34), pp.1–12.

Yalom, I. (2001) *The Gift of Therapy: Reflections on Being a Therapist.* London: Piatkus.

Yalom, I. (1980) *Existential Psychotherapy*. New York: Basic Books.

Yin, R. (2012) *Applications of Case Study Research.* Thousand Oaks, CA, London, New Delhi, Singapore: Sage Publications.

Yin, R. (2009) *Case Study Research: Design and Methods. Fourth Edition*. Thousand Oaks, CA: Sage Publications.

Yontef, G. (2002) The relational attitude in Gestalt therapy theory and practice. *International Gestalt Journal*, Vol.25(1), pp.15–34.

Zadra, J. & Clore, G. (2011) Emotion and perception: The role of affective information. *WIREs Cognitive Science*, Vol.2, pp.676–685.

Websites

Adamson, E. (2019) www.slam.nhs.uk/about-us/art-and-history/the-adamson-collection [Accessed online 21/08/2019].

Bartholomew, J. (2007) *Transitional Bodies Exhibition*. www.aic-iac.org/wp-content/uploads/Exhibition_Bartholomew3.pdf

British Association of Art Therapists (BAAT) Ethics and Art Therapy. www.baat.org/Membership/Documents/Professional-Advice

British Association of Art therapists (BAAT) (2004) About Art Therapy. www.baat.org/about-art-therapy

Kramer, E. (2004) *Art Tells the Truth*. (Film) Lenfim Studio. Accessed on 10/03/2017 at http://vimeo.com/33476299

Lester, S. (1999) *An introduction to phenomenological research*, Taunton: Stan Lester Developments. www.sld.demon.co.uk/resmethy.pdf [Accessed online 16/09/2020]

Ostrowska, A. (2013) Edward Adamson: Art as healing. *Wellcome Trust Library Blog*. http://blog.wellcomelibrary.org/2013/08/edward-adamson-art-as-healing/ [Accessed online 21/08/2019].

Plath, S. (1969) *Mushrooms*. https://allpoetry.com/poem/8498359-Mushrooms-by-Sylvia-Plath.

SLaM (2019) www.slam.nhs.uk/about-us/art-and-history/the-adamson-collection [Accessed online 21/08/2019].

Webster, C. (2006) *The Beautiful Women Project*, www.cherylannwebster.com/beautiful-women-project/).

Yarosh, D. (2019b) Why Luxury is Valuable: Status Aspirations and Self-Signaling Create Premium Value in Luxury Consumers Goods, pp.1–6. www.danyarosh.com/why-luxury-is-valuable.html

Index

Note: Page references in *italic* refer to figures, in **bold** to tables. Case studies by name are located under "research studies, participants". Case studies by topic can be found in brackets at the end of corresponding entries.

For Product Safety Concerns and Information please contact our EU representative GPSR@taylorandfrancis.com Taylor & Francis Verlag GmbH, Kaufingerstraße 24, 80331 München, Germany